Boundaries in Psychotherapy

Boundaries in Psychotherapy

Ethical and Clinical Explorations

Ofer Zur

American Psychological Association

Washington, DC

Published by
American Psychological Association
750 First Street, NE
Washington, DC 20002
www.apa.org

To order
APA Order Department
P.O. Box 92984
Washington, DC 20090-2984
Tel: (800) 374-2721; Direct: (202) 336-5510
Fax: (202) 336-5502; TDD/TTY: (202) 336-6123
Online: www.apa.org/books/
E-mail: order@apa.org

In the U.K., Europe, Africa, and the Middle East, copies may be ordered from
American Psychological Association
3 Henrietta Street
Covent Garden, London
WC2E 8LU England

Typeset in Palatino by Stephen McDougal, Mechanicsville, MD

Printer: Maple-Vail Book Manufacturing, Binghamton, NY
Cover Designer: Minker Design, Bethesda, MD
Technical/Production Editor: Tiffany L. Klaff

The opinions and statements published are the responsibility of the authors, and such opinions and statements do not necessarily represent the policies of the American Psychological Association.

Library of Congress Cataloging-in-Publication Data

Zur, Ofer.
  Boundaries in psychotherapy : ethical and clinical explorations /
by Ofer Zur. — 1st ed.
      p. cm.
  Includes bibliographical references and index.
  ISBN-13: 978-1-59147-737-2
  ISBN-10: 1-59147-737-9
  1. Psychotherapist and patient. 2. Psychotherapy—Moral and ethical aspects.
I. American Psychological Association. II. Title.
  [DNLM: 1. Psychotherapy—ethics. 2. Physician-Patient Relations—ethics.
3. Practice Management, Medical—ethics. WM 62 Z96b 2007]

  RC480.8.Z87 2007
  616.89′14—dc22   2006035436

British Library Cataloguing-in-Publication Data
A CIP record is available from the British Library.

Printed in the United States of America
First Edition

Important Notice

The statements and opinions published in this book are the responsibility of the author. Such opinions and statements do not represent official policies, standards, guidelines, or ethical mandates of the American Psychological Association (APA), APA's Ethics Committee or Ethics Office, or any other APA governance group or staff. Statements made in this book neither add to nor reduce requirements of the APA "Ethical Principles of Psychologists and Code of Conduct" (2002, see also http://www.apa.org/ethics/code2002.html), hereinafter referred to as the APA Ethics Code or the Ethics Code, nor can they be viewed as a definitive source of the meaning of the Ethics Code Standards or their application to particular situations. Each ethics committee or other relevant body must interpret and apply the Ethics Code as it believes proper, given all the circumstances. Any information in this book involving legal and ethical issues should not be used as a substitute for obtaining personal legal and/or ethical advice and consultation prior to making decisions regarding individual circumstances.

Contents

Preface

As a young child, I often pondered how we know if God exists. As a young man, I wondered why Jerusalem could not be peacefully shared by all religions. As a new oceanographer (one who studies saltwater, i.e., oceans) and limnologist (one who studies the life in freshwater, with a focus on lakes and ponds), I questioned why the oceans, which are almost 80% of the surface of our planet, are not used more efficiently for food production. As a young psychologist, I questioned whether it was true that men are inherently warlike and, likewise, what the role of women is in the making of wars. More recently, I have contemplated whether isolation and great privacy are necessary for physical, emotional, and spiritual healing. I imbibed questioning, pondering, and wondering with my mother's milk. In the early 1950s, my mother, also a psychologist, was already wondering about and advocating for Arab women's rights in Israel while my father focused on issues of justice for the poor. Dinners in my household, past and present, have not been about the "soup of the day" but the "idea of the day."

My penchant for questioning all things extends to my fascination with the nature, type, construction, dismantling, and permeability of boundaries—any kind of boundaries, human-made, natural, or God- or spirit-made boundaries. As a paratrooper in the Israeli Army, I experienced the boundaries of space and gravity. As a lieutenant and combat officer, I have stood on the boundary of life and death when my soldiers died in combat and I was wounded in the 1973 war. As an oceanographer and deep-sea diver, I passed through the boundary between air and water and then plumbed the boundless boundaries found everywhere in the depths of the seas. As a fish researcher in Africa, I encountered the human-made boundaries of civilization in remote parts of East and Central Africa. These days, as a psychologist, I am fascinated by therapeutic boundaries, both around the therapeutic relationships and between therapists and clients.

One of the inspirations for this book can easily be traced to the late 1980s, which is soon after I moved from the Berkeley/Oakland Bay Area to the small town of Sonoma in northern California. I received a call from a mother, whose kindergarten-age child was a classmate of one of my children, requesting to see me for an urgent couple therapy session. She told me that her husband, with whom I played pickup basketball, had suggested that she call me. She had found out that, at age 42 and already the mother of four, she was again pregnant, in the 2nd month, and needed to make an urgent decision about the pregnancy. Being trained psychodynamically in "city-centered therapy" and risk management practices, I told her such dual relationships were inappropriate and probably unethical. At this point, her husband joined us on the phone and, both obviously irritated with me, explained that they chose me *because* they knew me from the basketball court and from school and not from the Yellow Pages or other impersonal sources. In his attorney's voice, the husband explained to me that they chose me because they knew and trusted me and that confidence would speed up the process of deciding what to do about the pregnancy. Faced with their insistence and distress, I told them I would think about the matter and would get back to them by the next day. Several consultations with clinical, ethical, and legal experts clarified to me what I suspected: Treating people I know in the community is commonly regarded as a boundary violation, below the standard of care, and, most important, a very high risk from a risk management point of view. Remembering my years in Africa when people in need of help did not go three villages down the river to find a healer but chose the shaman in their own village, who knew them, their parents, and ancestors, I called back and told the couple that I would see them in therapy and do my best to help them come to a mutually agreed decision.

Moving to a small town brought me to the realization that people chose me *because* they knew and trusted me and that bumping into my clients outside the office would neither destroy the therapeutic alliance nor hurt therapy. In fact, as my friend and author, Sam Keen, insists and many of my clients agree, it may even help. At that time, there was very little in the literature to support this intuitive knowledge, and even less support was available from ethicists, attorneys, and risk management experts. As a result, I started conversing with the few like-minded professionals I could find and later started lecturing and publishing on the topic. In 2002, I coauthored (with Arnold Lazarus) *Dual Relationships and Psychotherapy*, the first comprehensive book that proposed a flexible, context-based look at dual relationships. During that same period and since, the American Psychological Association (2002; see also http://www.apa.org/ethics/) "Ethical Principles of Psychologists and Code of Conduct" evolved and now provides more flexible guidelines regarding dual relationships and bartering and, most important, stresses the importance of context in ethical decision making. Additionally, a few more articles and a number of books have been published with a new and refreshing view of boundaries, dual relationships, and therapy. However, there still seemed to be a vacuum—a need for a text that would include a flexible, context-based, and comprehensive look at various boundary issues, including nonsexual touch, self-disclosure, gifts, and home visits. My hope is to fill the vacuum, to satisfy that need, and, in one slim volume, to provide a broader view of therapeutic boundaries in all their diversity.

Acknowledgments

The act of writing this book on boundaries required me to cross many . . . boundaries. From concept to the first word, there were commonly held beliefs to be challenged, ethical interpretations to be braved, and invisible professional lines to be crossed. Then, as with any book, there were schedules to be followed and deadlines to be met with countless decisions and revisions—and finally the end of the road was reached. Across these boundaries and over hurdles, I was assisted every inch of the way by a coterie of extraordinary people. First and foremost, Lansing Hays of the American Psychological Association (APA) Books Department supported my writing of the book. I would like to give special thanks to the APA Books development editor, Susan Herman, who provided the most thorough and helpful feedback, assistance, and support an author could hope for, bringing the book to a higher level and all the way to the finish line. Special thanks are also given to APA Books production editor, Tiffany Klaff, who worked hard to help me express my ideas better and translate my Hebrish (Hebrew–English) to English. My friend and colleague Arnold Lazarus always provided an open and challenging mind, sharp editorial pen, and fearless encouragement to explore the nature and utility of boundaries. My longtime friend and personal editor, Mimi Capes, began editing my work 30 years ago, when I was an oceanographer, deep-sea diver, and fish-farming researcher exploring the boundaries of the ocean and seeking a boundless source of nourishment for all humankind, and she continues to do so today. Nola Nordmarken was instrumental in reflecting on interpersonal boundaries in the chapter on touch and the family–work boundaries in the home office chapter. She also provided much valuable feedback for several other chapters. One of the inspirations for my general work on dual relationships and this book came from relentless challenges from my friend and colleague, Sam Keen, regarding the sometimes unquestioned assumptions and boundaries of psychotherapists. Finally, my beloved wife, Jennifer, provided me with tender care and limitless support during the writing of this book. My gratitude to all of these people is without bounds.

Boundaries in Psychotherapy

Introduction

Boundaries, in general, have multiple meanings and implications and therefore have been defined, discussed, and applied differently by different people in different situations. Many definitions focus on geographical or political boundaries, such as borders between regions, territories, countries, or continents. Then there are biological boundaries, such as the skin or various internal membranes. The laws we live by are boundaries, too; they articulate the limits of legally accepted behaviors. Still other boundaries are more abstract, such as social, racial, interpersonal, interpsychic, and spiritual boundaries. Depending on how one defines and draws them, boundaries can separate or unite, enhance or deplete, help, heal, or harm. What unifies all the definitions of boundaries is the essential aspect that they differentiate between two or more physical–actual or elusive–abstract entities.

Boundaries in therapy are extremely important because they define the therapeutic–fiduciary relationships. They distinguish psychotherapy from social, familial, sexual, business, and many other types of relationships. Originally, the impetus to define and articulate clear and distinct therapeutic boundaries came from the desire to enhance therapeutic effectiveness by creating a protective "frame" around the therapeutic exchange and also from the wish to protect clients who may become vulnerable during the process of therapy.

Since the inception of psychotherapy, the field has struggled with the definition and application of boundaries. Clinicians tend to intuit what boundaries mean, but explaining and using them in practice is often challenging. This book intends to shed light on the definition and use of psychotherapeutic boundaries. Different orientations and different eras have thought of, defined, and implemented boundaries differently. While some clinicians emphasize the importance of clearly defined and consistently used boundaries, others stress the therapeutic importance of dismantling certain boundaries. Psychoanalysis differentiates between external boundaries around the therapeutic relationship and between clients and analysts as well as internal boundaries between the ego and the repressed unconscious. Family therapists have concentrated on the meaning, quality, and functionality of boundaries between subsystems and members within families and the nature of the boundaries around families. Cognitive–behavioral therapists focus on the boundaries and relationships between people's cognition, affect, and behavior. Feminist therapists look critically at the meaning of economic, social, and moral boundaries between men and women and between social and economic classes. Humanistic–existential therapists concentrate on interpersonal boundaries, whereas transpersonal and spiritual therapists direct their attention to spiritual boundaries. Most broadly, the field has looked at the ever intangible and ever mysterious boundaries between body, mind, and spirit.

This book provides a probing, inclusive discussion of boundaries, their ethics, and their clinical utility. Its purpose is to help the reader identify boundaries in therapy and to differentiate between boundary crossings and boundary violations. For example, readers will gain new knowledge and strategies for distinguishing among multiple relationships that are unavoidable, whether inconsequential or helpful, and those that are exploitative. This book leads the reader through analyses of the many types of boundaries in psychotherapy and outlines how to navigate these complexities in ethically and clinically appropriate ways. Although I discuss the clinical efficacy of many boundary crossings, the book clearly states that sexual relationships between therapists and clients are counterclinical, unethical, and often illegal. In addition, there are many other nonsexual situations in which certain questionable behaviors become clear boundary violations: for example, accepting inappropriate expensive gifts or large sums of money, or practicing extensive and improper self-disclosure for the sole benefit of the therapist.

Boundary Crossing Versus Boundary Violation

There are two types of boundary activity in psychotherapy: boundary violations and boundary crossings. A *boundary violation* occurs when a therapist crosses the line of decency and integrity or misuses his or her power to exploit or harm a client. Boundary violations usually involve exploitative business or sexual relationships. And, as stated earlier, boundary violations are always unethical and are likely to be illegal (Gabbard & Lester, 1995; Gutheil & Gabbard, 1993; Williams, 1997). Boundary crossings are very different from boundary violations; they are more elusive and much harder to define. Most broadly, *boundary crossing* refers to any deviation from the strictest professional role (Gutheil & Gabbard, 1998; Knapp & Slattery, 2004) or from traditional, hands-off, "only-in-the-office," "no self-disclosure" forms of therapy or departure from risk management procedures (Lazarus & Zur, 2002). Boundary crossings can be part of well-constructed treatment plans designed specifically to increase therapeutic effectiveness. The most obvious and most common boundary crossings are self-disclosure, the exchange of small gifts or greeting cards, nonsexual touch (Pope, Tabachnick, & Keith-Spiegel, 1987), incidental encounters outside the office (Sharkin & Birky, 1992), and home visits (Morris, 2003). Boundary crossings are often an integral part of behavioral, cognitive–behavioral, humanistic, existential, group, or feminist therapy. Some boundary crossings, such as incidental encounters between therapists and clients outside the office, are neither planned nor are part of the treatment plan.

Two Types of Boundaries for Psychotherapy

Because what constitutes a boundary in therapy varies among practitioners and orientations, its definition becomes difficult. Like Langs (1982), D. Smith and Fitzpatrick (1995) discussed boundaries in terms of "a therapeutic frame, which defines a set of roles for the participants in the therapeutic process" (p. 499). The frame is described as including structural elements such as the place where therapy occurs, the duration and time of therapy, and fee agreements. It also includes concerns with confidentiality, which is the protective layer around the therapeutic exchange. These boundaries are articulated in state and federal laws, professional codes of ethics, and the informed consent or professional contract between therapist and client. For example, laws governing the practice of psychotherapy define the therapeutic relationship as a fiduciary or contractual relationship of special trust in which confidentiality is maintained and in which therapists assume certain responsibilities for their clients, which are not a part of everyday relationships.

Boundaries of another sort are drawn between therapist and client rather than around them. In line with this definition, Gutheil and Gabbard (1993) regarded boundaries as the "edge" of appropriate behavior. Such behavior might include therapist self-disclosure, making or allowing contact outside of the normal therapy session, giving and receiving gifts, and regulating physical proximity of therapist and client during sessions. Although maintaining the therapeutic frame as well as these more interpersonal boundaries is the prime responsibility of therapists, clients cocontribute and codefine the nature and development of therapeutic boundaries (Knapp & Slattery, 2004).

Both types of boundaries determine the nature of the therapeutic relationship while marking what is included or excluded. Boundaries can be viewed as membranes—sometimes rigid, thick, and impenetrable; other times flexible, thin, and permeable. Perhaps an even more apt simile for the purposes of this book would be to say that boundaries are like walls: human-made constructs that can be erected or dismantled and allow for the addition of gates, doors, or barriers.

Crossing Boundaries While Meeting the Standard of Care

Since its inception, the field of psychotherapy has wrestled with the relationships between boundary crossing and the standard of care as manifest in such issues as touch, self-disclosure, gifts, and dual relationships. As early as 1931, a prescient Sigmund Freud, in a poignant and amusing letter to Sandor Ferenczi, a prominent psychiatrist and member of his inner circle, was one of the first to recommend adherence to a certain standard with regard to the boundary issue, in this case, of touch. Ferenczi made no secret of the fact that he kissed his patients and let them kiss him, a detail that distressed and troubled his mentor. Freud did not hesitate to draw the line when he wrote to Ferenczi on December 13, 1931:

> Now picture what will be the result of publishing your technique. There is no revolutionary who is not driven out of the field by a still more radical one. A number of independent thinkers in matters of technique will say to themselves: why stop at a kiss? Certainly one gets further when one adopts "pawing", as well, which after all doesn't make a baby. (E. Jones, 1957, p. 175)

To this day, psychotherapists are still struggling to identify a unified and generally accepted professional standard of care with regard to boundaries.

The standard of care is one of the most important concepts in mental health. It has been described as the qualities and conditions that prevail, or should prevail, in a particular mental health service, and that a reasonable and prudent practitioner follows. It guides clinicians by providing a minimum standard and is the basis for malpractice suits and discipline by licensing boards. Although of high importance, the standard of care in psychotherapy—especially with regard to therapeutic boundaries—is not easily defined and is a dynamic standard that changes and evolves with time. Generally, the standard of care is derived from the following sources: laws or statutes, licensing boards' regulations, case law, ethical codes of professional associations, consensus of professionals, and common practices within the community (Appelbaum, 1993; Caudill, 2004; Doverspike, 1999; Gutheil, 1998; Woody, 1988). When it comes to therapeutic boundaries, it is not a completely objective or yardstick-type standard that can be found in textbooks. It is a rather subjective standard that is determined by a variety of factors, such as the setting in which therapy takes place, the therapeutic modality, and the client factors.

Oddly enough, the standard of care is ultimately determined by the judges and juries who rely on the testimony of experts, who very often provide conflicting testimonies because of the fact that they are hired by opposing parties in civil, administrative, or criminal disputes. It seems that beyond a basic agreement to do no harm; to eschew exploitation of clients; and to respect clients' autonomy, dignity, and privacy; there is very little agreement as to what falls within the standard and what does not.

The vagueness of the standard with regard to therapeutic boundaries has resulted in broad disagreements and deep controversies around the issues of boundaries. Because the standard is based on what is "reasonable" and is based on community standards, it is open to interpretation and debate, varying according to situations, settings, cultures, localities, therapists, philosophies of treatments, and clients. The following are a couple of examples illustrating the complexities involved in determining the standard of care in psychotherapy with respect to boundaries.

A home visit with a mentally ill, elderly, bed-bound client who is in need of psychiatric care is likely to fall within the standard of care. However, the same home visit with an able, borderline client who highly sexualizes her relationship with her therapist and is likely to need firm and clear therapeutic boundaries would fall below the standard of care. Similarly, having a toddler sit on the therapist's lap during family therapy may be reasonable but certainly is not the case with an adult.

There are other variances. Significant self-disclosure is likely to be an important and integral part of humanistic, feminist, or group therapy. Therefore, these types of therapy fall within the standard of care if they are used for clinical reasons and are designed to enhance authentic relationships that will benefit clients. However, similar self-disclosure is most likely viewed to fall below the standard by an analytically oriented psychotherapy, as it is likely to interfere with transference analysis. Dual relationships in military settings—in which the therapists and clients are also comrades-in-arms—are legally mandated and thus fall within the standard of care even though they may involve conflicts of interest (see this chap. 1, this volume, p. 29–31). However, business dual relationships with obvious conflicts of interest are likely to fall below the standard of care. Extensive appropriate touch by Reichian or other body-oriented psychotherapists clearly falls within the standard of care. However, excessive and repeated touch by most verbally oriented psychotherapists may not fall within the parameters of the standard. Deliberately harming or exploiting clients and sexual relationships with clients always fall below the standard of care. Consultation with experts is one of the best ways to establish that the standard of care was met (Younggren & Gottlieb, 2004). Such consultations with experts allow the psychotherapist to demonstrate that the boundary crossing or dual relationship he or she engaged in is reported to be similar to what other reasonable psychotherapists would do under similar circumstances.

Toward the end of the 20th century and the beginning of the new millennium, there have been two significant and contradictory forces that have affected the relationships between boundaries and the standard of care. On the one hand, the emergence of risk management concerns during this period has shifted the interpretation of the standard of care somewhat toward a more cautious position. In terms of boundaries, the shift is toward more formal relationships in which practices such as touch, gifts, walks outside the office, or dual relationships are considered more conservatively. On the other hand, there has also been a significant increase in the number of publications that link boundary crossings to the most commonly practiced theoretical orientations, review their potential clinical benefits, and discuss the inevitability of boundary crossing, including dual relationships, in many communities and settings (e.g., Barnett & Yutrzenka, 1994; Lazarus & Zur, 2002; Schank & Skovholt, 2006; Williams, 1997, 2003; Zur, 2000). These two forces have been operating simultaneously and pulling the standard of care in two opposing directions. On the one hand, the proliferation of risk management practices leads to more practitioners practicing defensively, which in turn creates a new, generalized standard. On the other hand, the emergence of a more open approach in professional publications and more flexible codes of ethics tilt the standard toward a more flexible, context-based standard.

Crossing Boundaries While Managing Risk

In light of the great increase in medical malpractice suits and licensing boards' litigation in the 1990s, risk management practices have assumed increasing importance. Such new developments have an obvious impact on the application of most boundaries in psychotherapy. There are several influences that have caused the increased focus on risk management. Insurance companies have an interest in reducing civil litigation and jury verdicts. Licensing boards and other consumer protection agencies have also been promoting risk management practices to increase protection and safety for consumers. Clinicians are highly motivated to avoid licensing board investigations and sanctions and are naturally eager to avoid malpractice suits. It is understandable that risk management's primary focus has been on boundary issues, especially sexual boundary violations.

In psychotherapy, risk management generally refers to the practice of minimizing risk to clients and psychotherapists. It usually involves risk identification, risk assessment, risk analysis, and risk control. In principle, it is, indeed, important to manage risk to both clients and psychotherapists (Bennett, Bryant, VandenBos, & Greenwood, 1990; Doverspike, 2004). Reducing the risk to clients is an ethical and professional commitment articulated in the American Psychological Association's (APA, 2002; see also http://www.apa.org/ethics/) "Ethical Principles of Psychologists and Code of Conduct" (hereafter referred to as the APA Ethics Code) and almost all other codes, under the general principle of nonmaleficence, or "do no harm." More specifically, it is the therapists' clinical, ethical, and legal obligation to minimize the risk of clients who are mentally ill hurting themselves or others. Similarly, it is the therapist's professional and ethical obligation to minimize risk and harm to abused partners and children and any client who is in harm's way. Equally appropriate is the therapist's commitment to reduce physical, emotional, professional, or financial risk to herself or himself.

Risk management is similar to what has been called *defensive medicine*. There is a debate in the field of medicine, in general, and specifically in mental health as to whether risk management practices are primarily aimed at protecting the practitioners or the consumers. Taking a pragmatic and widely accepted approach, Gutheil and Gabbard (1993) and Williams (1997, 2003) defined risk management in realistic terms as the course whereby therapists refrain from implementing certain interventions because they may be misinterpreted, questioned, or frowned on by boards, ethics committees, or courts. Topping the list of risk management behaviors to be avoided are boundary crossings and dual relationships, which include gifts, touch, and barter (Woody, 1988, 1998). The aim, according to this most popular understanding of risk management, is to prevent or preemptively defend the health care provider against lawsuits, criminal charges, allegations by licensing boards, or complaints by ethics committees. Preventive medical risk management practices have also resulted in a significant increase in the cost of care and may possibly compromise the quality of care.

From a clinical point of view, this approach to risk management practices can affect the quality of care negatively (Gutheil & Gabbard, 1998; Lazarus, 1994; Zur, 2005a). Examples include therapists who may choose to not touch a distressed patient, refuse a gift from a child, avoid a potentially helpful self-disclosure, or refuse to leave the office with a client to help him or her overcome a social phobia. From a service point of view, some risk management advice may leave some segments of the population untreated. Following the more conservative risk management injunction never to leave the office, for example, would mean more bedridden or housebound clients without access to in-person psychotherapy. A refusal to barter might equate to denial of service to a potential client who is cash poor. If all therapists avoided all dual relationships, many people in rural and other small communities would have no access to psychiatric and psychotherapeutic care.

This book asserts that risk management and quality psychotherapeutic care are not mutually exclusive, and the protection of clients can be achieved simultaneously with the protection of the practitioners. Doverspike (2004) described this ideal goal in which "Reasonable clinicians protect themselves by protecting their patients" (p. 210). The challenge is to find ways to practice ethically with a responsible, clinical foundation while protecting clients and therapists from risk. To achieve this goal one must follow an ethical approach to risk management practices based on the loftiest clinical and ethical principles. This includes treating clients with respect and dignity; honoring clients' autonomy and privacy; and intervening according to the client's problems, personality, culture, gender, situation, and so on. As articulated in chapter 4 of this volume, a thorough and well-documented decision-making process, treatment plan, and clinical records, and, when necessary, consultations, referrals, and signed informed consents are likely to simultaneously increase the quality of care and provide protection to clinicians.

Boundary Shifts in the History of Psychotherapy

Paradoxically, Freud, who laid the foundations for strict, analytically based, therapeutic boundaries, crossed many of them himself. He gave some of his patients gifts, provided financial support to several others, entered into a matchmaking arrangement with two of his clients, gave legal advice to some, and offered a meal to the patient known as the Rat Man. Melanie Klein and Freud both analyzed their clients during their vacations and crossed the professional–familial line by analyzing their own children. Winnicott, like Ferenczi, touched his clients, and Carl Jung engaged in a sexual dual relationship with his patient, Sabina Spielrein, who was not only his patient and lover but also his student and colleague (Gutheil & Gabbard, 1993; Kerr, 1993).

However, concerns with therapeutic boundaries came to the forefront of the field only after Gestalt therapy, with Frederick Perls at the helm, became enormously popular during the sexual revolution of the 1960s. Manifest sexual and other boundary violations were openly espoused at Esalen Institute in California, where therapists and clients often became playmates and even lovers. In response to the sexually and other permissive attitudes of the 1960s and 1970s, there was pressure on psychology, in general, and on psychotherapy, in particular, to articulate and provide more specific guidelines regarding therapists' conduct vis-à-vis their clients. As a result, consumer protection agencies, licensing boards, and legislators joined ethicists and psychotherapists in establishing clear restrictions with regard to therapist–client sexual dual relationships (Gutheil & Gabbard, 1998). Therapists were instructed not only to resolutely avoid sexual relationships but also to make every effort to avoid any kind of dual relationship. The increasingly litigious culture of the 1980s and thereafter, as well as the increased focus on risk management in medicine, led to more spoken and unspoken injunctions against any deviation from hands-off, only-in-the-office, "no self-disclosure" therapy. Barter, gifts, nonsexual touch, and dual relationships were generally viewed as hazards from a risk management standpoint.

The early 1990s witnessed a slight shift in professional attitudes to psychotherapeutic boundaries. There was a growing acknowledgment that boundary crossing, such as nonsexual touch and self-disclosure, can be clinically helpful, and nonsexual dual relationships were unavoidable under some circumstances, for example, in rural areas, small towns, military settings, and among constituents of distinct individual communities, such as churches, the deaf, gay men and lesbians, and other minorities (e.g., Barnett & Yutrzenka, 1994; Field, 1998; Lazarus, 1994). Partly in response to this growing awareness, the APA (1992), National Association of Social Workers (1996), and other professional associations revised their codes of ethics, particularly with regard to dual relationships. They all presented a clear recognition of the fact that dual relationships are neither always avoidable nor always unethical.

From the mid-1990s to the present time, the debate on the utility and ethics of therapeutic boundaries has intensified. On one side of the debate, consumer protection agencies, licensing boards, risk management experts, many ethicists, and psychoanalytically oriented therapists continue to advocate clearly defined and distinct boundaries around the therapeutic relationship and between therapists and clients (Epstein, 1994; Gabbard & Lester, 1995; Pope & Vasquez, 2001; Syme, 2003; Woody, 1988). The clergy's sexual abuse scandals have lent support to the notion that clients need protection from exploitative priests, psychotherapists, and other authority figures (Rutter, 1989). On the other side of the debate, there have been a growing number of ethicists and professionals who point out that flexible boundaries can be clinically helpful when applied ethically (e.g., Barnett, 1999; Helbok, Marinelli, & Walls, 2006; Herlihy & Corey, 2006; Knapp & VandeCreek, 2006; Lazarus & Zur, 2002; Nickel, 2004). Additionally, there have been a growing number of publications that discuss the fact that nonsexual dual relationships are neither always avoidable (Canter, Bennett, Jones, & Nagy, 1996; Nagy, 2005; Schank & Skovholt, 2006) nor always unethical or harmful and, in fact, can be clinically beneficial (Barnett, 1999; Corey, Corey, & Callahan, 2003; Ebert, 1997; Gabriel, 2005; Herlihy & Corey, 2006; Kessler & Waehler, 2005; Lazarus, 1998; Moleski & Kiselica, 2005; Schank & Skovholt, 2006; Williams, 1997; Younggren & Gottlieb, 2004; Zur, 2004b).

Boundaries and the Codes of Ethics

The codes of ethics are one of the most important resources for defining and guiding the therapeutic encounter. As such, they articulate the boundaries around and within the therapeutic relationship. Although the term *boundaries*, as it is used in this book, almost never appears in any of the major professional organizations' codes of ethics, the codes clearly define the parameters of psychotherapeutic boundaries. The codes give us guidance with regard to what kind of behaviors, values, and attitudes are appropriate within the therapeutic frame (i.e., what should be included or excluded by therapeutic boundaries). Although the term *boundaries* may not often appear in the codes, the concern with boundaries is nevertheless implicit and paramount. It manifests itself in the sections of the codes relating to informed consent, limits of confidentiality, disclosures, fee agreements, third-party payments, scopes of practice, and boundaries of competency, all of which ultimately define the therapeutic frame and create the outer limits around the therapeutic encounter. Other sections in the codes of ethics such as those concerning therapists' power, exploitation, conflicts of interest, and sexual and nonsexual dual relationships, inform us of the nature and quality of the boundaries between, rather than around, therapists and clients.

The codes of ethics of psychotherapists' professional associations, such as the APA, American Psychiatric Association, National Association of Social Workers, National Board of Professional Counselors, and American Counseling Association, have evolved through the years alongside cultural and professional changes that reflect the increasing awareness and knowledge of the field. Like most other codes during the mid-20th century and ensuing decades, the APA Ethics Codes have been nonspecific and have concentrated on the general ideas of promoting client welfare and discouraging abuse of power by therapists. Partly in response to the sexually and other permissive attitudes of the 1960s, especially in the human potential and humanistic movements in California, there was pressure on psychology and counseling, in general, and psychotherapy, in particular, to articulate and provide more specific guidelines with regard to therapists' conduct vis-à-vis their clients. The sexually "liberated" culture of the 1960s helped focus the APA Ethics Codes of 1977 and 1981 on restricting sexual touch of clients by therapists and social and sexual dual relationships between therapists and clients (Lazarus & Zur, 2002). Therapists were instructed not only to resolutely avoid sexual relationships but also to make every effort to avoid any kind of dual relationship. In the late 1980s and 1990s, awareness extended among ethicists that earlier versions of the APA Ethics Code had set too low a threshold for acceptable dual relationships. Partly in response to the growing awareness and acceptance of unavoidable dual relationships, many professional associations (e.g., APA, 1992; National Association of Social Workers, 1996) revised their codes of ethics in clear recognition of the fact that dual relationships are neither always avoidable nor always unethical (Williams, 1997). All these professional associations' codes, including other codes, such as the National Board for Certified Counselors (2005a) acknowledge that some dual relationships are unavoidable and advise therapists to refrain from entering into a dual relationship if it could reasonably be expected to impair therapists' objectivity or effectiveness or risk exploitation or harm to clients.

The APA Ethics Code of 2002 has taken another step forward in bringing flexibility to boundaries in psychotherapy as manifested in three sections. First, in its "Introduction and Applicability" section, it provides a clarification and an explanation of some of the modifiers that are used in the code (e.g., *reasonably, appropriate, potentially*). More specifically, it states, "As used in this Ethics Code, the term *reasonable* means the prevailing professional judgment of psychologists engaged in similar activities in similar circumstances, given the knowledge the psychologist had or should have had at the time" (APA, 2002, p. 1061; see also http://www.apa.org/ethics/code2002.html#intro [para. 6]). This later clarification is likely to establish the fact that the ethics of therapeutic boundary crossing and dual relationships are primarily determined by the contexts of therapy (i.e., client, setting, therapy, and therapist; see chap. 3, this volume) rather than by an arbitrary standard that fits all situations. Second, the 2002 APA Ethics Code moved further away from the clear denouncement that bartering is unethical, which appeared in the earlier codes, by dropping the strongly cautionary language of the 1992 code with regard to bartering. Third, the code took one more step with regard to context-based evaluations of dual relationships when it added this statement, "Multiple relationships that would not reasonably be expected to cause impairment or risk exploitation or harm are not unethical" (APA, 2002, p. 1065; see also http://www.apa.org/ethics/code2002.html#3_05). Similarly, the American Counseling Association (2005) significantly revised its code of ethics in 2005 to include the statement that "potentially beneficial" dual relationships are not unethical.

In summary, none of the professional organizations' codes directly refer to boundary considerations such as self-disclosure, gifts, nonsexual touch, home visits, home office, and so on. Most of them provide a cautionary statement regarding dual relationships, but none of them denounce them as unethical. The principles of beneficence (benefit) and nonmaleficence (no harm), fidelity and responsibility, integrity, justice, and respect for people's rights and dignity that are embraced by all the codes cover the concern that all boundaries in therapy are used with these principles in mind.

Map of the Book

I use the term *client* to represent the word *patient*, both meaning any consumer of psychotherapeutic services. Similarly, I use the terms *therapy* and *psychotherapy* interchangeably, meaning counseling and services by mental health professionals. Also, when I use the term *dual relationships*, I also mean *multiple relationships*.

Part I, Boundaries in Context, provides a wide-ranging view of boundaries in therapy. Chapter 1, "Dual Relationships," defines and describes different types of dual relationships as they take place in different settings such as rural, isolated, and close-knit communities; college and university campuses; professional training institutes; and other settings. Chapter 2, "Reflections on Power, Exploitation, and Transference in Therapy," takes a critical look at issues such as power, the "slippery slope" (i.e., when innocent boundary crossings lead to boundary violations), and transference. Chapter 3, "Contexts of Therapy," articulates the four factors that constitute the context of therapy: client factors, setting of therapy, therapy factors, and therapist factors. Chapter 4, "A Decision-Making Process for Boundary Crossing and Dual Relationships" explains in detail an ethical decision-making process that involves critical thinking and risk–benefit analysis.

Part II, Boundaries Around the Therapeutic Encounter, deals with issues that affect the therapeutic frame. Chapter 5, "Time and Money," attends to issues of management of time, fees, billing, and bartering. Chapter 6, "Space for Therapy," speaks of the clinical and ethical complexities involved in providing services outside the office, which include home visits, adventure therapy, and attending ceremonies, among others. Chapter 7, "The Home Office Practice," discusses clinical, ethical, and safety considerations involved in conducting therapy from one's own home. Chapter 8, "Telehealth and the Technology for Delivering Care," covers a wide range of cutting-edge topics related to new technologies, such as psychoeducation, e-therapy, technology-mediated therapy, and other technology-assisted alternatives to face-to-face therapy.

Part III, Boundaries Within the Therapeutic Encounter, explores the types of boundaries that exist between therapists and clients. Chapter 9, "Self-Disclosure," discusses the ethical, clinical, and contemporary technological considerations involved in self-disclosure. Chapter 10, "Touch in Therapy," identifies the wide range of benefits and concerns that can arise from nonsexual touch. Chapter 11, "Gifts," discusses the ethical and clinical complexities involved in giving, receiving, or rejecting gifts. Chapter 12, "Personal Space, Language, Silence, Clothing, Food, Lending, and Other Boundary Considerations," attends to these rarely considered issues.

Part IV, Final Thoughts, provides a summary of the book. Appendix A provides a quick reference guide to the differences between boundary crossing and boundary violations. Appendix B presents direct quotes from the different professional associations' ethics codes on boundaries and dual relationships.

I

Boundaries in Context

1

Dual Relationships

The term *dual relationship* in psychotherapy refers to any situation in which multiple roles exist between a therapist and a client (Bennett, Bryant, VandenBos, & Greenwood, 1990; Koocher & Keith-Spiegel, 1998; Pope & Vasquez, 2001). This book uses the more popular term *dual relationship* to discuss dual and multiple relationships. Dual relationships can be social–communal (when a client is also a friend, social acquaintance, fellow congregation member, or works at the store where the therapist shops), sexual (when a client is also a lover), business (when a client is also a business partner), professional (when a client is also a professional colleague), or familial (when a client is also a family member).

It is important to differentiate between boundary crossings such as therapeutic touch, clinically driven self-disclosure, home visits, and gift exchanges, which do not entail a secondary relationship and those associations that involve dual relationships. Therapists in the former situations operate exclusively in their clinical capacity and, therefore, these situations are not considered dual relationships. For the same reasons, attending a client's wedding or self-disclosing for clinical reasons rather than social ones does not constitute social or other dual relationships. However, if self-disclosure or attending the client's wedding takes place in the course of a social relationship or as part of a community relationship between the therapist and client, it constitutes a dual relationship (Lazarus & Zur, 2002). Incidental, chance encounters between therapists and clients outside the therapy room that are not part of a social, collegial, or business connection do not constitute dual relationships. Unlike most bartering for goods, bartering for services—such as when a client paints a therapist's home, fixes his or her car, or cleans his or her office in lieu of payment—inherently creates a secondary business association and, therefore, is a dual relationship (Zur, 2004a).

Thus, it is clear that whereas all dual relationships are boundary crossings, not all boundary crossings are dual relationships. Exploitative or harming dual relationships are unethical boundary violations because they harm clients and violate the most basic ethical and moral mandate to avoid harm. Sexual relationships and exploitative business relationships with active clients have been cited as the most common and serious examples of such boundary violations (Bersoff, 1999; Gutheil & Gabbard, 1993; Herlihy & Corey, 2006; Knapp & VandeCreek, 2006; Koocher & Keith-Spiegel, 1998; Lazarus & Zur, 2002; Pope & Vasquez, 2001; Reamer, 2001). Appropriate, unavoidable, mandated, clinically enhancing dual relationships or those that are a normal part of small communities are boundary crossings.

Dual relationships can be simultaneous or sequential. Simultaneous dual relationships are those relationships that take place at the same time as therapy is taking place. Examples are when a therapist and client attend the same church services or play on the same athletic team while therapy is taking place. Sequential dual relationships are those that follow one another. Examples are when a former fellow student starts therapy after graduation or when therapist and client decide to enter into a social relationship after therapy has ended (DeJulio & Berkman, 2003; Gabriel, 2005; Herlihy & Corey, 2006; Lazarus & Zur, 2002; Reamer, 2001).

Dual relationships can also be differentiated by the degree of involvement or engagement between clients and therapists (e.g., Helbok, 2003; Kitchener, 1988; Schoener, 1997; Younggren & Gottlieb, 2004). Attending the same community event such as the Sunday sermon or Little League game, implies less intimate involvement than working side by side on a fundraiser, which, in turn, is less intimate than an ongoing social relationship. Similarly, there is a difference between therapist–client relationships that have developed in the context of long-term, intensive psychotherapy and less intimate or shorter duration activities such as biofeedback, brief therapy, and assessment.

Rural and Isolated Communities

Rural or small, isolated communities present psychotherapists who practice there with a wide range of unavoidable dual relationship situations that are embedded in the social structure and therefore become normal, accepted, and expected (e.g., Barnett & Yutrzenka, 1994; Campbell & Gordon, 2003; DeJulio & Berkman, 2003; Gabriel, 2005; Hargrove, 1986; Helbok, Marinelli, & Walls, 2006; Herlihy & Corey, 2006; Schank & Skovholt, 1997, 2006; Simon & Williams, 1999; Sleek, 1994; Stamm, 2003; Stockman, 1990). People in such communities are familiar with most of their fellow citizens, including the local therapists. These communities often offer only a limited pool of therapists from which to choose. As a result, therapists and clients often know each other prior to the start of therapy and interact with each other in a number of nonclinical capacities before, during, and after therapy. These interactions may include the therapist and client chaperoning their children on class trips, serving on some local committees together, coaching in the same league, belonging to the only health club in town, shopping at the same market, and attending the same church and community events. They may engage in unavoidable business dual relationships, for example, when a therapist buys a car from a client's local car dealership, which is the only one in town, or shops at a client's grocery store. There will be all types of social and professional dual relationships with local professionals. Local attorneys, physicians, business owners, pastors, dentists, machinists, judges, and policemen very often socialize, entertain, or serve alongside the people they serve or do business with. Therapists are no exception (Faulkner & Faulkner, 1997; Helbok, 2003; Moleski & Kiselica, 2005; Nickel, 2004; Schank & Skovholt, 1997, 2006; Zur, 2000). Multiple relationships are the manifestation of the interdependence and interconnectedness that are not only characteristic of such communities but, in fact, essential to their integrity, survival, and prosperity.

Practically speaking, solo practitioners in such small communities cannot avoid interacting with their clients at the local market, community events, or school functions. Avoiding all nontherapy contacts would require the therapists to lead the life of hermits (Helbok et al., 2006; Younggren & Gottlieb, 2004). If therapists choose to isolate themselves, they may be looked on with suspicion by members of such communities who rely on familiarity for the development of trust (Moleski & Kiselica, 2005; Zur, 2000).

Close-Knit Communities

Similar to the isolated, rural communities are the small, close-knit communities that exist within large metropolitan areas (Schank & Skovholt, 2006). These include church, synagogue, and other spiritual communities (Geyer, 1994; Llewellyn, 2002; Montgomery & DeBell, 1997); Hispanic, African American, American Indian, Chinese, and other ethnic communities (Kertész, 2002; Sears, 1990); gay male, lesbian, and bisexual communities (Kessler & Waehler, 2005; A. J. Smith, 1990); deaf and other disabled communities and the recovery communities (Guthmann & Sandberg, 2002; Zur, 2000), among others (Gabriel, 2005; Helbok et al., 2006). What is unique about these communities, besides their size, is their membership's strong sense of affiliation and equally strong feelings of interdependence, mutuality, and affiliative philosophy. The bonds among members in these communities make them highly cohesive and, to varying degrees, separated from other communities or even isolated from the world around them. Some of these communities have a legitimate sense of being shunned, misunderstood, or even persecuted by the society at large, which in turn increases their sense of cohesion and self- or mutual reliance. The self-reliance aspects are tied to the sense of survival and are often manifested in members exclusively seeking help and guidance within the community rather than from the outside. Along these lines, clients are likely to deliberately and systematically seek therapists who share their cultural heritage, spiritual or religious orientation, language, history, values, disability, or sexual orientation.

Christian fellowship members may choose their pastors or other church leaders as their psychotherapists because they have heard their Sunday sermons; know their spiritual, communal, and familial values; have witnessed them leading prayer groups; and have watched them interact with members of the congregation (Geyer, 1994; Llewellyn, 2002; Montgomery & DeBell, 1997). Gay male or lesbian clients often choose gay male or lesbian therapists in their community who are "out" and whom they know share their subcultural background or difficult experiences in a generally homophobic and often discriminatory culture (Kessler & Waehler, 2005). Clients who are deaf often seek deaf therapists in their communities whom they know personally, whom they respect or have seen overcome difficulties related to impairment or discrimination. Additionally, deaf clients are likely to choose therapists who can sign to avoid the use of interpreters. These therapists tend to be hearing impaired themselves and are often involved in the deaf community (Guthmann & Sandberg, 2002). Jewish, African American, or Hispanic clients may seek familiar therapists with similar cultural or ethnic backgrounds from within their own community who share their heritage, values, language, or customs (Lazarus & Zur, 2002). A newly "clean and sober" member of the Alcoholics Anonymous fellowship may seek a therapist who is part of the local fellowship and with a similar cultural and socioeconomic background who has been clean and sober for a long period of time (Doyle, 1997; Moleski & Kiselica, 2005; Zur, 2004b).

Many of the previously mentioned clients in these communities choose their therapists because they are familiar, because they respect and appreciate their background, values, and conduct. Anonymity is not valued in many of these cultures, whereas familiarity is highly valued. As a result, therapists in these communities often have multiple, primarily social, relationships with their clients. The emphasis on self-reliance and mutual dependency within these communities often leads to therapist–client business dual relationships as well.

College and University Campuses

At college and university counseling centers that are located on campuses, where the therapists are very likely to run into their clients frequently, incidental encounters are indeed common and dual relationships, consequently, may arise. Because many therapists in these counseling centers are graduate students themselves, they may often interact with other students, including their clients, in various capacities. Many scenarios are possible: attending classes, lectures, graduation ceremonies, concerts, parties, and sports events; participating in team sports or frequenting the campus health club or pool together; both working part time at a library or a research center (Hayman & Cover, 1986; Hyman, 2002).

More clinically complex and potentially unethical dual relationships occur when clients attend classes that are being taught or assisted by their therapists. Sometimes neither therapist nor client is aware of the situation in advance, but then again, they may be. The situation can be avoided if clients can switch to other classes than those taught by their therapists. However, if the client must take a class at a specific time and there is no alternative class or the therapist cannot back out of the assignment, the situation may be unavoidable. Clients who like and appreciate their therapists may intentionally choose to attend classes taught by them. However, faculty members must be sensitive to their conduct with regard to students and address this type of situation with supervisors and university administration in a manner that protects the student's privacy and welfare. The difficulty of such dual relationships can arise from different sources. One important concern is that the therapists, in their teaching capacity, are also evaluating or grading the student–clients, a predicament that can involve a conflict of interest that may interfere with the therapeutic process. For example, a low grade given by a therapist–teacher to a client may result in the client resenting and distrusting the therapist. Conversely, therapists who like their clients are likely to grade them more favorably in the classroom setting.

College and universities are expected not only to educate but also to professionally and socially mentor young people and help them with the transition to adulthood. Some of the complications of dual relationships on college and university campuses arise precisely from these expectations. Therapists, who may be professors, teaching assistants, or students, and who are inherently also mentors, may find themselves wearing several hats with their clients. Navigating among these different roles and avoiding harming conflict-of-interest situations is a constant challenge for therapists on college campuses. It is interesting to note that exploitative relationships are rarely reported at college and university counseling centers (Gallagher, Gill, & Sysco, 2000). The reasons for the low reporting rate may vary from the fact that abuse is rare to the feeling of community that is characteristic of college campuses to the power differential between students and instructors that can cause reluctance on the part of the student to file complaints for fear of retaliation.

Professional Training Institutes

Training institutes such as psychoanalytic or Jungian training institutes, or various humanistic, cognitive–behavioral, or family therapy training establishments, present unique and complex dual relationship situations. Like supervisors, analysts, and instructors in these institutions, the trainees and candidates also tend to be licensed professionals with graduate degrees. Naturally, these institutions attract people who share their appreciation of a certain philosophy, theoretical orientation, or even worldview. The trainees in these places are neither necessarily young nor necessarily professionally inexperienced and, in fact, often are seasoned professionals who seek advanced or more focused professional training.

The first training institutes were the psychoanalytic institutes in Europe and the United States in the first part of the 20th century. Their tradition still seems to be influential in many analytic, Jungian, and similar training establishments. In this tradition, trainees are mandated to undergo analysis with one of the senior training analysts on staff. These senior training analysts may also serve as instructors of case conferences, mentors, class instructors, and even supervisors or members of the committee evaluating the trainees' progress and readiness for graduation. Needless to say, these multiple therapeutic, supervisory, and evaluative relationships are highly complex and fraught with abundant potential for conflicts of interests (Pepper, 1990; Schoener, 1997; Wakefield, 1996).

The most cited concern is whether the trainees are willing to be honest and open in therapy knowing that their senior training analysts also serve on the committee that evaluates them. Other boundary issues surface because most institute staff and trainees have been involved with each other in some capacity such as supervision, analysis, mentoring, evaluation, case conference, and so on. As a result, these analytic societies have developed a reputation for being entangled with one another rather incestuously (Wakefield, 1996). The scope of the multiple relationships in training institutions extends beyond the therapeutic and didactic realms. D. H. Lamb, Catanzaro, and Moorman (2004) reported that 32% and 45% of therapists reported discussing potential new social relationships with former clients and supervisees, respectively. Trainees often go to the professional conferences, serve on committees and task forces, and attend retreats and other social gatherings alongside their therapist–analyst supervisors, mentors, and those who evaluate their progress. The fact that like-minded people are drawn to these institutions and that trainees are often as old and as experienced professionals as their training staff seems to increase the possibility of not only ideological compatibility but also emotional and physical attraction. As a result, the inherent professional and social dual relationships that are as complex as they are prevalent in these settings often spill over into intimate and sexual relationships as well.

Boundary problems plagued the early psychoanalytic institutions and have been the focus of several exposé-type books and articles. Grosskurth's (1991) book, *The Secret Ring: Freud's Inner Circle and the Politics of Psychoanalysis,* and Kerr's (1993) book, *A Most Dangerous Method,* are among the many works that detail some of this history. Far from the idea of the analyst as a blank screen espoused by Freud and his students, these early analysts practiced a wide range of boundary crossings and boundary violations, as mentioned previously. Most notable are Jung, Karen Horney, Stekel, and others, who allegedly had sexual relationships with their clients. Freud and Melanie Klein psychoanalyzed their own children, Ernest Jones had Klein analyze his children and wife, and there were many in the early analytic circles who analyzed each other's family members, mistresses, and so on. Ferenczi analyzed the daughter of the woman he was having an affair with and then fell in love with the girl. While at the University of Toronto, Ernest Jones became the subject of an allegation of sexual involvement with a client whom he attempted to pay to keep quiet about the matter. Frieda Fromm-Reichmann has written that her husband, Erich Fromm, was a patient when they became romantically involved. Otto Rank reportedly became sexually involved with a former patient. Freud himself encouraged a young analyst whom he was treating to follow his instincts and divorce his wife so he could marry a patient. Freud was reported to have had financial motives in this case, hoping for a donation to the psychoanalytic movement from the patient's wealthy family.

Mandated Dual Relationships in Military and Prison Settings

Military and the prison–police systems are examples of settings or institutions that by law require all psychotherapists who work within them to be continuously involved in dual relationship situations. What is unique about these two governmental structures is the fact that the psychotherapists' primary allegiance is to the institutions rather than to their clients. Military law mandates that military psychologists give higher priority to national defense, unit integrity, and combat readiness than to concerns with the welfare of the individual psychotherapy client (Johnson, 1995; Staal & King, 2000). Similarly, forensic psychotherapists who work in prisons and jails must give higher priority to matters of security than to concerns with the welfare of their individual clients. Police psychology also presents a complex and often unavoidable multiple relationship situation in which the psychologists may be concurrently involved in training, fitness-for-duty evaluations, consultation, hostage negotiation, and other roles (Zelig, 1988). These psychotherapists are employed by a city, county, state, or federal government, so needless to say, these mandated priorities often put them in difficult conflict-of-interest situations in which they may need to act in a way that may harm the client but serve the institution.

A very particular kind of community can be found on small islands or heavily guarded military bases in foreign countries.

The ultimate inaccessible and remote setting is that of an aircraft carrier. In this distant, confined, and highly regimented environment, therapists sleep, eat, play, conduct drills, undergo medical exams and drug testing, and entertain with, next to, or close to their past, current, and future clients (Johnson, Ralph, & Johnson, 2005). Gonzalez, a naval officer and psychologist, describes his experience right after September 11, 2001:

> When our unit was mobilized a short time later, my patients and I became shipmates: the office was replaced with a ship and the couch with bunks. We were no longer doctor and patient, but comrades in arms with the common goal of national defense. (Zur & Gonzalez, 2002, p. 315)

Active duty, military, clinical psychologists or psychiatrists fulfill dual roles as commissioned military officers and therapists or clinicians. In addition to these dual roles, therapists also have dual agency, bearing responsibility for and loyalty to their therapy clients as well as the military or the Department of Defense (DOD; Hines, Adler, Chang, & Rundell, 1998). Johnson (1995) described military psychologists as "serving two masters." In fact, by military law, DOD is the therapists' legally defined client rather than the individual in the consulting room. Additionally, commanders have the authority to assign individuals under their command to seek mental health services or undergo an evaluation in accordance with military regulations (Staal & King, 2000). The result of such regulations is that military therapists have neither control over whom they consult or evaluate nor ways to prevent dual relationships and conflicts of interest. Military psychologists may find themselves in a perplexing conflict-of-interest situation in which they are mandated to evaluate their commander or superior for fitness for duty (Zur & Gonzalez, 2002). Because of the inherent duality in the military, informed consent should always be used. Clients in these settings must be fully informed of the potential eventualities that they may face as a result of engaging in a dual relationship; and, when possible, therapists can leave it to clients to decide if they want to engage in the dual relationship.

The focus of military and penal institutions on security and safety has resulted in laws that mandate therapists to cross the line of confidentiality in certain situations. Military law has the "need to know" clause, which refers to the right of a commanding officer to view or be privy to specific client information that is relevant to national security or combat readiness. Military psychologists, in fact, serve also as the DOD's gatekeepers, being required to divulge private and sensitive information to superiors if it has a bearing on national defense and unit integrity (Johnson, 1995). Similarly, psychotherapists in prisons are part of the prison staff and, as such, are first and foremost concerned with issues of security. Any information that is revealed during psychotherapy sessions that may have bearing on security and safety must be reported to the prison authority. As members of the prison staff, therapists may be mandated to serve also as guards or even armed guards. As in the military, these dual roles can lead to ethical and clinical convolutions and conflict of interest, which therapists in the conventional therapeutic world seldom encounter.

Financial Dual Relationships

Therapists loaning money to clients and clients loaning money to therapists are additional, potentially troublesome boundary issues. Unlike loaning a client a small sum for a bus or subway fare at the end of a session, loaning a significant sum involves a business or financial dual relationship. Similarly, receiving loans from clients constitutes a business dual relationship that can be extremely complicated, possibly leading to a conflict-of-interest situation, impaired judgment, and interference with the clinical process. Psychologists reported in one survey that they "rarely" lent money to clients (D. H. Lamb & Catanzaro, 1998; Pope, Tabachinick, & Keith-Spiegel, 1987) and viewed it as basically unethical (DeJulio & Berkman, 2003). The problem with significant loans comes from the possibility that the party receiving the loan or gift may feel indebted to the loaning party. This applies to loans from therapists to clients or from clients to therapists. The loaning party may feel imposed on, taken for granted, or exploited; unhappy with how the loan was given or the terms of the gift–loan; or resent not being paid back on time. Therapists making loans to clients can easily create a sense of obligation, and when exploitation takes place, it is a boundary violation. Therapists receiving loans from clients, regardless of how wealthy they are, may be construed as exploitation and misuse of power and, therefore, a boundary violation.

As often is the case with our forefathers and prominent figures in our profession, although clearly concerned with boundaries, Freud nonetheless provided some clients with "extensive financial support" (Gutheil & Gabbard, 1993, p. 189), including financial support to the Wolf Man (Isaac, 2004). When a therapist refers, introduces, or directs a client to a third party to receive a loan, this constitutes a business dual relationship if the therapist and the third party have a business relationship. Similarly, if a client refers a therapist to a third party for a loan, it may also constitute a business dual relationship if the client and the loaning party have a business relationship. Either way, therapists are advised to be very cautious in such situations and make sure that they do not exploit, harm, or clutter up the therapeutic relationship by adding such complicated and potentially emotionally loaded transactions.

Buying goods from clients or selling goods to clients is another boundary consideration because it creates relationships secondary to the therapeutic one. This practice is very common among acupuncturists, chiropractors, nutritionists, and holistic health practitioners. A survey of psychologists revealed that about a quarter of the surveyed psychologists might engage in selling a product to a client under some circumstances, and more than half would consider buying goods from clients (Borys & Pope, 1989). A more recent survey reveals that almost all (94%) social workers stated that selling a product to a client is either never ethical or ethical only under rare conditions (DeJulio & Berkman, 2003). As with any boundary crossing, borrowing from, lending to, buying from, or selling to clients must be conducted with sensitivity and great care that these practices are neither exploitative nor obstructive to the therapeutic process. At all times the welfare of the client must be held paramount.

Referrals

Referrals are the lifeline of psychotherapists, whether they practice privately or as part of a clinic or even an institution. Referrals of new clients to therapists can come from different sources: directories such as online or Yellow Pages; current or former clients; clients' family members, friends, or colleagues; therapists' family members, friends, or colleagues; or attorneys, teachers, or business acquaintances. The referrals can be self-referred as well. Referrals that bear on the existing psychotherapeutic relationships by introducing new elements fall under the heading of boundary crossing. Dual relationships may be established when the current client has a relationship with the new referral, which means that the therapist has dual loyalties to two associated clients. From an ethical and boundary point of view, the concern about referrals is whether the subsequent introduction of the new therapeutic relationship affects the existing therapeutic relationship and in what ways (Shapiro & Ginzberg, 2003).

Referrals are sometimes similar to gifts. When it comes to referrals, the intent and the meaning of the individual making the referral as well as the therapist who receives the referral determines its appropriateness. If the referral creates indebtedness, the therapist may face a conflict of interest in which clinical decisions and the welfare of the client may become secondary to pleasing or fulfilling the expectations or even demands of the referral source. If a therapist accepts a referral that is likely to lead to a conflict of interest or loss of objectivity, it is unethical and a boundary violation, unless the acceptance of the referral is mandatory. As with gifts, the intent and the meaning of the person making the referral, as well as the therapist who receives the referral, would determine a number of things. It would reveal the nature, quality, and magnitude of the impact of the referral, or secondary therapeutic relationship, on the original therapeutic relationship and between the referral source and the receiving therapist (see chap. 11, this volume). Although most referrals by clients or their family members or friends are boundary crossings, boundary violations occur in situations in which therapists solicit referrals from clients that are clearly motivated by their need or greed, or put them in compromising conflict-of-interest positions that are likely to impair their clinical judgment and harm the original or new clients.

Among the richest resources for referrals in the private practice setting are referrals from satisfied current or former clients. There can be many reasons for clients to refer family members, friends, and colleagues to their therapists. The satisfied customer may refer with the hope that the person referred will get the help that the client received. It may be driven by the hope that the therapist may help the client's spouse, partner, parent, or child and thereby help the client, too. If clients believe their therapists to be in financial need, they may give referrals to help them out. It can also be a way to show off their therapists to others. Or perhaps clients cannot draw healthy and appropriate boundaries with friends and relatives, and the referral becomes a power play to level the playing field and even create indebtedness. Of course, the character of the relationship between the referring client and the newly referred one is very important in determining the propriety of seeing the referred client in therapy. For example, if a client has a stable, long-term relationship with the person he or she refers to his or her therapist, the referral may be appropriate. However, if the relationship between the referring client and referred person is volatile or conflict ridden, accepting the new referral is likely to interfere with the primary relationship. In the latter case, it is inappropriate to accept the referred client because it is likely to create a conflict of interest or conflict of loyalty on behalf of the therapist. As with gifts, therapists and clients can discuss the intent, meaning, and potential impact of the referral.

There are several concerns with referrals from clients. If the therapist accepts such referrals, the original client or the new one may later feel that the therapist favors one over the other. If one client tells secrets about the other, the therapist may be caught in a triangle, which may then compromise confidentiality or quality of treatment. If the therapist feels indebted to the client, it may impair clinical judgment. Shapiro and Ginzberg (2003) raised the concern that such referrals may result in ethical conflicts such as exploitation, dual relationships, and sacrifice of confidentiality. Similarly, Epstein and Simon (1990) suggested that taking a referral from a client is a form of exploitation in that the therapist receives more than just the fee in compensation for treating the client. Another matter worthy of thought is how accepting a referral from a former client may affect the client's decision to return to treatment in the future (Gabbard & Pope, 1989). Bartering for client referrals is unethical, and most ethics codes bar therapists from "kickback"-type compensation for referrals. This would also be a boundary violation and exploitative dual relationship and likely to impair the therapist's clinical judgment and exploit the client.

Colleagues and friends of therapists are another important source of referrals and, potentially, a flattering one that also creates a dual relationship situation. Therapists must be clear about the bounds of confidentiality and especially about what can be communicated to the referral source regarding the client. Divulging confidential information to colleagues or other referral sources about clients has been cited as one of the most common transgressions therapists unethically and, in most situations, illegally commit (Shapiro & Ginzberg, 2003; Sharkin, 1995). The therapist must also watch for a sense of inappropriate indebtedness to the colleague or friend and whether the referral had a negative impact on their relationship. They also have to assess whether a conflict of interest arises, because therapy may reveal some unflattering or even dangerous aspect of the colleague's or friend's nature that could leave the therapist in an awkward position of dual loyalty.

Therapists referring a client to a spouse, family member, or anyone who is closely related to the therapist should be cautious. For example, if there are other options, it is ill advised to refer a client to a dentist or car mechanic who is also the spouse of the therapist because it is likely to create imprudent dual relationships and a conflict-of-interest situation (Behnke, 2006) that may well constitute a boundary violation. However, sometimes such referrals are unavoidable, as may be the case in a small, isolated community in which the referring therapist's spouse is the only nutritionist or chiropractor in the area. Generally, any referral by the therapist that can benefit him- or herself should be fully disclosed and discussed with the client and avoided if it is done primarily for the benefit of the therapist rather than the client. Informing the client of the relationship to the therapist does not necessarily reduce the risk of exploitation and harm. Failure to inform the client of such relationships is a boundary violation and betrayal of trust.

Self-referrals are another important source of clients. Almost all advertisements are geared to tapping this source of clientele. Self-referred clients can become a boundary and dual relationship issue if they are, for example, friends of the family, neighbors, or fellow congregation members. As was discussed earlier, familiarity and self-referrals are unavoidable and a normal part of rural, ethnic, spiritual, disabled, and many other close-knit and interdependent communities. Therapists can find themselves in an uncomfortable situation if they realize, after therapy starts, that a self-referred client has an intimate, antagonistic, or otherwise complex relationship with another existing client. The situation may be complicated, may often involve conflict of loyalties, and can be fraught with difficulties, loss of objectivity, or reduced clinical efficacy, whether only one or both of the clients are aware of the situation. In this instance, the prudent practitioner should seek a consultation, go through a thorough and well-documented ethical decision-making process, and document the decision process.

Coauthors' or Collaborators' Dual Relationships

A singular and rarely mentioned type of dual relationship occurs when therapists and clients write a book or an article, cocontribute to a project, or perform together. The best-known example is Yalom's collaboration with his client, Elkin, on their bestseller about her therapy, *Every Day Gets a Little Closer* (Yalom & Elkin, 1990). Similar collaborations have taken place when therapists and clients collaborate on a research project or are involved in any other artistic or other project together.

Ethics of Dual Relationships

Unlike the general guidelines provided for most other boundary crossings, the APA Ethics Code and other such codes provide specific guidelines regarding dual relationships. In addition to the codes of ethics, other publications during the 1980s and early 1990s focused primarily on the risks of dual relationships and their association with sexual boundary violations (e.g., Borys & Pope, 1989; Epstein, Simon, & Kay, 1992; Gutheil & Gabbard, 1993; Kitchener, 1988; Pope, 1989, 1990a; Pope, Sonne, & Holroyd, 1993; Simon, 1991, 1994; Sonne & Pope, 1991; Strasburger, Jorgenson, &

Sutherland, 1992). A shift took place in the mid-1990s that has continued through the early years of the 21st millennium.

In the late 1980s and 1990s, there was growing awareness that nonsexual dual relationships were unavoidable under some circumstances such as in rural areas and the military. During the shift in the 20th century, mentioned previously, more publications have reviewed the inevitability and potential clinical utility of dual relationships (e.g., Barnett, 1999; Campbell & Gordon, 2003; Ebert, 1997; Hedges, Hilton, Hilton, & Caudill, 1997; Herlihy & Corey, 2006; Kessler & Waehler, 2005; Lazarus, 1994, 1998; Lazarus & Zur, 2002; Reamer, 2001; Tomm, 1993; Williams, 1997; Zur, 2000, 2001b, 2004b, 2005a). Thus, Younggren and Gottlieb (2004) wrote the following:

> Professional practice abounds with the potential for multiple relationships, and the circumstances under which these types of relationships occur are quite varied. Although psychologists frequently choose to enter into these types of relationship, many may actually be unavoidable, and in some situations one can even conceptualize the avoidance of the dual relationship not only as unethical but as potentially destructive to treatment itself. (p. 255)

The APA (1992), National Association of Social Workers (1996), and other major professional associations revised their codes of ethics to reflect wider acknowledgment of the fact that dual relationships are neither always avoidable nor always unethical. All these codes advised therapists to refrain from entering into a dual relationship if it could reasonably be expected to impair their objectivity or effectiveness or risk exploitation or harm to clients. The 1990s and the early 2000s were also marked by an intensification of the debate around dual relationships. The interlocutors were those who focused on consumer protection and risk management and those who asserted that some dual relationships are unavoidable, benign, a normal and healthy part of close-knit or small communities, and can be clinically beneficial. As a result, the 2002 APA Ethics Code added the sentence, "Multiple relationships that would not reasonably be expected to cause impairment or risk exploitation or harm are not unethical" (p. 1065; see also http://www.apa.org/ethics/code2002.html#3_05). It then also took an important step to align the code of ethics with the standard of care by clarifying the term *reasonable*. This emphasized that the appropriateness of dual relationships is to be judged in the context of therapy rather than by some abstract, arbitrary yardstick (Younggren & Gottlieb, 2004; Zur, 2004b). Similarly, the American Counseling Association's (2005; see also http://www.counseling.org/Resources/CodeOfEthics/TP/Home/CT2.aspx) Code of Ethics declared that dual relationships that are "potentially beneficial to the client" (p. 5) are not unethical (Herlihy & Corey, 2006). Also, the National Board of Certified Counselors (2005a) acknowledges that some dual relationships are unavoidable.

To sum up the codes of ethics of all major professional organizations as they relate to dual relationships in psychotherapy, I emphasize the following: (a) Nonsexual dual relationships are neither always avoidable nor always unethical; (b) sexual dual relationships with present and almost all former therapy clients are always unethical; (c) terminating therapy to pursue sexual relationships is unethical; (d) sexual relationships with recently terminated clients is unethical and the APA Ethics Code specifies a 2-year minimum wait, which has often been adopted by other organizations; (e) therapists must be aware of their influential power over their clients and never use this power to exploit or harm them nor to benefit the therapist at the expense of the client; and (f) therapists must try to avoid conflict-of-interest situations and those dual relationships that could reasonably be expected to impair their judgment and objectivity, interfere with performing therapy, evaluation, or supervision effectively, or harm or exploit patients. (Note to item d: Even beyond the 2-year minimum, therapists are advised to either avoid or be extremely cautious with regard to sexual relationships with former clients.)

Dual Relationships in the Context of Therapy

The meaning and effect of dual relationships on the therapeutic process can only be understood within the context of therapy. As discussed in chapter 3, the context of therapy involves four factors: client factors such as age, culture, presenting problems, and history; setting factors such as rural or urban, solo private practice or hospital setting; therapy factors, including theoretical orientation and length, type, and quality of therapeutic relationships; and, finally, therapist factors such as age, culture, gender, training, and scope of practice.

The client's culture, maturity, and presenting problem are probably some of the most important factors determining the appropriateness of establishing a dual relationship with a client. A professional or social dual relationship with a healthy and mature client may be appropriate whereas the same relationship will be highly disruptive to therapy with a client with paranoid or borderline personality disorder (Lazarus & Zur, 2002). Also, clients with a long history of physical or sexual abuse, with sensitivity to boundary considerations, may be less likely to benefit from dual relations as they cross traditional boundaries and may be experienced as betrayal or violation. On the one hand, some clients from certain cultural or political backgrounds may even expect some level of duality, as may be the case with American Indian, Latino, feminist, or gay male and lesbian clients (Gabriel, 2005; Zur, 2000). On the other hand, dual relationships with clients who tend to sexualize relationships or those who are paranoid, volatile, obsessively jealous, psychotic, or present borderline personality disorder features are clinically and ethically ill advised.

In addition to what was previously noted, there are numerous settings in which client–therapist interactions are mandated (e.g., military, prisons), unavoidable (e.g., rural and isolated communities), or normal and expected (e.g., ethnic minority, church, gay and lesbian, and disabled communities; Gabriel, 2005; Helbok, Marinelli, & Walls, 2006; Schank & Skovholt, 2006). In contrast, dual relationships are less common in many private practices in metropolitan areas. They are also counterindicated in inpatient and hospital settings or as part of psychiatric emergencies units (Younggren & Gottlieb, 2004).

The therapeutic modality is another highly relevant factor in determining the appropriateness of establishing dual relationships with clients. Humanistic psychotherapy emphasizes the importance of authentic and congruent relationships between clients and therapists and, therefore, is likely to endorse nonsexual and nonexploitative dual relationships because they are likely to enhance such authentic relationships (Jourard, 1971b). Along these lines, Williams (1997) stated, "Nothing in the theory of behavior therapy would or should preclude socializing with patients" (p. 244). Many feminist therapists support any therapist–client interactions that reduce the traditional doctor–patient power differential and increase familiarity and connectivity (Feminist Therapy Institute, 1987; Greenspan, 1995; Herlihy & Corey, 2006). Similarly, behavioral, cognitive, family, and culture-sensitive therapists do not exclude dual relationships when they are likely to enhance therapeutic outcome or are not likely to hurt it (Lazarus & Zur, 2002). Analytically oriented therapists who emphasize maintaining the analyst's anonymity and keeping the therapeutic boundaries clear, consistent, and distant obviously are not likely to endorse any form of dual relationships (Epstein & Simon, 1990; Langs, 1982; Simon, 1991).

The nature of the therapeutic alliance is another important determining factor in the decision of whether to engage in a dual relationship. Obviously, trusting and positive therapeutic relationships between therapists and clients are more compatible with dual relationships than distrustful or hostile relationships. Similarly, a short-term relationship or when the therapist serves primarily as an educator is less likely to create unpredictable complexities in the "nonclinical" relationship than long-term therapy or therapy that focuses on transference analysis.

Therapists' factors also play a role in the decision of whether to engage in dual relationships. Generally, therapists who are more communally oriented or come from a highly communal culture (e.g., Latino, Jewish, etc.) tend to be more open to dual relationships with their clients than those who come from more individualistic, Northern European cultures, who tend to focus on personal space and privacy (Lazarus & Zur, 2002). Therapists' training and socializing into the profession are likely to affect their openness to such relationships. Those whose training was analytically focused are less likely to view dual relationships as appropriate or beneficial than those whose training was humanistic, feminist, or cross-cultural. Similarly, therapists whose training emphasized risk management are more likely to avoid dual relationships, when possible, compared with therapists who were trained in rural areas or in more flexible, context-based ethics (Williams, 1997; Zur, 2005a).

Informed Consent

Discussing the issues of dual or multiple relationships with clients is of extreme importance. Regardless of whether the dual relationships are mandatory, unavoidable, or elective, therapists must obtain an informed consent from their clients regarding the nature of the dual relationships and the risks and benefits involved in entering into such relationships (Herlihy & Corey, 2006; Younggren & Gottlieb, 2004). If necessary, exit strategies should be discussed and agreed on. Obviously, each setting would require a different type of discussion and different type of consent. In settings in which dual relationships are mandatory, unavoidable, or likely, the informed consent must be presented prior to the first session and should be discussed with clients before treatment gets under way.

The following is a sample of an informed consent that is focused on small-town dual relationships.

Dual relationships: Dual relationships (or multiple relationships) in psychotherapy refer to any situation in which therapists and clients have another relationship in addition to that of therapist–client, such as a social or business relationship. Not all dual relationships are unethical or avoidable. Therapy never involves sexual or any other dual relationship that impairs Dr. XX's objectivity, clinical judgment, or therapeutic effectiveness or can be exploitative in nature. Dr. XX will assess carefully before entering into nonsexual and nonexploitative dual relationships with clients. XX is a small community in which many clients know each other and Dr. XX. Consequently, you may encounter someone you know in Dr. XX's waiting room or Dr. XX out in the community. Dr. XX will never acknowledge working with anyone without his/her written permission. Many clients chose Dr. XX as their therapist because they knew him/her before they entered into therapy with him/her and/or because they are aware of his/her stance on the topic of dual relationships. Nevertheless, Dr. XX will discuss with you, his/her client/s, the often-existing complexities, potential benefits, and difficulties that may be involved in such relationships. Dual or multiple relationships can enhance therapeutic effectiveness but can also detract from it, and often it is impossible to know that ahead of time. It is your responsibility to communicate to Dr. XX if the dual relationship becomes uncomfortable for you in any way. Dr. XX will always listen carefully and respond accordingly to your feedback and will discontinue the dual relationship if he/she finds it interfering with the effectiveness of the therapy or the welfare of the client, and, of course, you can do the same at any time.

To Dual or Not to Dual:
How to Decide About Dual Relationships

A few decision-making models and guidelines have been developed for dual relationships (e.g., S. K. Anderson & Kitchener, 1998; Gottlieb, 1993; Kitchener, 1988). Most of these models focus primarily on power differential, potential for harm, and risk management considerations and imply that it may be best to avoid dual relationships, if and when possible. Additional, more flexible, and more applicable guidelines are provided by Barnett (1999), Ebert (1997), Herlihy and Corey (2006), Moleski and Kiselica (2005), Younggren and Gottlieb (2004), and Lazarus and Zur (2002). Partly based on these models and guidelines, the following is a more inclusive approach to dual relationships that acknowledges that some dual relationships are unavoidable but also views dual relationships as a healthy aspect of certain small and interdependent communities and, as such, potentially able to enhance trust between therapists and clients, therapeutic alliance, and clinical outcome. This approach comprises eight sets of questions.

First, are the dual relationships avoidable–elective or mandated–unavoidable? Also, are they expected, normal dual relationships or rare and unique within the communal context in which they take place? Dual relationships in the military are unavoidable. They are common, expected, and difficult to avoid in small, rural communities but are less common and avoidable in large, metropolitan areas where there is a wide selection of available therapists. Dual relationships in the gay male and lesbian or deaf communities, for instance, are avoidable but common and often expected.

Second, are there laws, regulations, or ethical guidelines that pertain directly to the dual relationship under consideration? Dual relationships in the military are legally mandated. Obviously, sexual relationships with clients are always unethical and are illegal in most states. Some codes of ethics, states' laws, and states' licensing boards limit the type of bartering therapists are allowed to engage in, whereas others define the parameters of dual relationships allowed in certain forensic situations.

Third, what is the nature, quality, and intensity or frequency of the dual relationship? Is it a personal, professional, or business dual relationship, and will the two parts of the relationship be implemented simultaneously or sequentially? For example, a dual relationship with a fellow congregation member whom you see infrequently at a Sunday mass is considered a simultaneous, social, dual relationship of low level of engagement.

The fourth set of questions involves four closely related questions, which make up the risk–benefit analysis: (a) What are the potential risks of entering into a dual relationship? (b) What are the potential benefits of entering into the dual relationship? (c) What are the potential risks of not entering into the dual relationship? and (d) What are the potential benefits of not entering into the dual relationship? This step involves an analysis of the likely consequences of engaging in a dual relationship, as well as the likely consequences of not engaging in a dual relationship with this particular client at this particular time and in a certain setting. The potential for conflict of interest, likely conflict of loyalties, and loss of objectivity must be seriously considered as this can have a significant negative impact on the therapeutic process. Also, it is very important, at this stage, to evaluate what might be the potential impact on the community. Part of the analysis must look at the compatibility between the two roles—therapeutic and nontherapeutic—that therapists may play. Several types of dual relationship (i.e., business, social, collegial) and level of engagement (i.e., intense, cordial, remote) may be an option, and in this case each option should be evaluated separately for its risks and benefits. Similarly, simultaneous versus sequential dual relationships should also be considered. Avoiding risk–benefit analyses and exclusively focusing on potential harm and risk management considerations would result in ignoring the potential benefits and advantages of dual relationships. Even mandatory dual relationships should be carefully assessed for their potential impact on the clinical work. Obviously, the risk–benefit assessment must take into consideration the contexts of therapy (i.e., client factors, setting, therapy and therapist factors), as detailed in chapter 3 of this volume.

The fifth set of questions involves the use of consultations: Does the complexity of the proposed dual relationship necessitate the use of a clinical, ethical, or legal consultation? Therapists must differentiate between these three different domains and employ an expert consultant accordingly. Rather than consulting with a clinician who practices down the hall, it is preferable to seek out an expert (Younggren & Gottlieb, 2004) or peer consultation. Therapists should engage a consultant when there is a risk that they may not be able to sustain clinical objectivity or may enter into conflict-of-interest situations.

The sixth set of questions involves the clients: Has the client been fully informed of the risks and benefits entailed in engaging in dual relationships? Similarly, has the client given an informed consent to the dual relationship, and is the client aware of possible consequences and (mentioned next) exit strategies? What are the client's reactions, responses, or input to the risks and benefits with which he or she was presented?

The seventh set of questions is related to change of plans and exit strategies: If the dual relationship turns out to negatively affect the client or the therapeutic work, what are the exit strategies, and what are the likely consequences of using them? Human relationships are often unpredictable, and dual relationships that seem initially to enhance the clinical process may affect it negatively later on. If a dual relationship proves harmful, an exit strategy must be constructed, discussed, and implemented. For example, seemingly benign and common social dual relationships in a tight lesbian community may turn competitive, possessive, fraught with jealousy, and highly disruptive to the therapeutic process. Therapists should weigh the options of disengaging from the social or the therapeutic relationships and discuss these options with the clients, including the possibility of referrals, before finalizing them. Consultations with an expert when dual relationships go sour are highly advisable.

The eighth set of questions involves the evaluation of the effect of a dual relationship: What tools and approaches must the therapist use, after the initial engagement, to continuously evaluate the effect of the dual relationship on the clinical work? Undoubtedly, eliciting a client's assessment of the situation is part of a therapist's determination of the appropriate application of the dual relationship.

Risk management has been central to dual relationship issues. Several authors have articulated risk management strategies for dual relationships (Gutheil & Gabbard, 1993; Herlihy & Corey, 2006; Koocher & Keith-Spiegel, 1998; Pope & Vasquez, 2001; Younggren & Gottlieb, 2004). This book takes the position that a thorough and well-documented decision-making process and treatment plan, clients' informed involvement in the decision-making process, and consultation, when necessary, is the best practice and thus the best risk management strategy.

The process of deciding to engage in dual relationships should be documented and placed alongside the treatment plan in the client's records. The records should reflect the client's participation in the decision-making process and, when necessary, should include a written and signed informed consent, a description of consultations, an exposition of the nature and type of the dual relationships, and, when applicable, referrals made. The decision-making process should show that the relevant client's factors, setting factors, therapy factors, and therapist's factors have been considered (see chap. 3, this volume). For detailed steps on ethical decision making regarding dual relationships in psychotherapy, see Figure 1.1.

Ultimately, the therapist must evaluate the actions she or he has decided on and ensure that they are consistent with the standard of care or with what should be expected from the average professional in the same or similar circumstances. However, periodical assessment and reassessment and corresponding adjustments of the course of treatment are also extremely important. Thus, by not etching the course of action in stone and maintaining a certain fluidity, therapy and the client–therapist relationships can remain in balance.

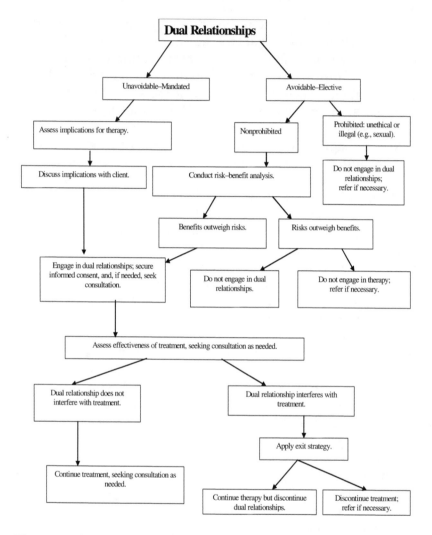

Figure 1.1. Dual relationships decision tree: Seeking consultation can be done at any point in the process.

2

Reflections on Power, Exploitation, and Transference in Therapy

This chapter discusses three of the most commonly raised and closely related points regarding boundaries in therapy. The first one is that given the power differential between therapists and clients, crossing therapeutic boundaries can lead to exploitation and harm of clients by their therapists. The second is the "slippery slope" phenomenon, which is the basis for an assertion that minor, and seemingly harmless, boundary crossings are likely to lead to harmful boundary violations. The third is the premise that boundary crossings are likely to interfere with transference analysis and muddle the transferential relationships.

Power and Boundaries

The major concern with boundary crossing in therapy is the power differential between therapists and clients and how therapists may use or abuse this power. Therapists are hired for their professional expertise, which consequently gives them an expert-based power over their clients (Frank, 1973). Therapists' seeming aura of wisdom also translates into a power advantage over their clients. Additionally, many clients seek therapy at times of crisis; others are anxious or depressed, which makes them inherently more vulnerable, augmenting the power differential between their therapists and themselves. Pope and Vasquez (2001) identified several types of power that pertain to therapists. These include power conferred by the state, power to name and define, power of testimony, power of knowledge, and power of expectation. This power differential has been described as one of the most important factors in determining the risk of harm to clients when therapists engage in boundary crossing (Kitchener, 1988). It was also listed as the first dimension in the decision-making model for avoiding exploitative dual relationships in therapy (Gottlieb, 1993).

Whether it is power derived from the state as manifested through licensing or the power emanating from therapists' knowledge, education, and expertise, they all give therapists the power to influence clients. As a result, therapists' suggestions, opinions, advice, or instructions are likely to be taken seriously by many clients, especially the ones who are more vulnerable to such influences. Such influence places the burden of responsibility not to abuse or exploit this power squarely on the therapist.

As noted, the power differential enables therapists not only to help and assist but also to exploit and harm their clients. The concern with therapists' power has been focused on therapists' using boundary-crossing interventions or on entering into dual relationships. Similar to the slippery slope idea, worries arise that an authoritative clinician or counselor who crosses boundaries and ventures beyond the threshold of only-in-the-office, hands-off therapy may foster sexual and other forms of exploitation. The proposed solution for the power differential problem is similar to the proposed solution for the slippery slope issue: avoidance, when possible, of all boundary crossing, and dual relationships, in particular. Some authors (e.g., Gonsiorek & Brown, 1989) have taken the subject of power a step further and suggested that "Once a client, always a client," meaning that therapists' power and potential to exploit and harm, especially in long-term psychotherapy, may last long after therapy and perhaps in perpetuity.

In the power differential argument against boundary crossing, clients are often portrayed as passive and malleable, even defenseless, perceiving their therapists as strong and superior (Lazarus, 1994; Tomm, 1993; Williams, 2002; Zur, 2000). In reality, many therapists work with clients who are much more powerful than they. Some clients are CEOs of large corporations, judges, power-house attorneys, master mediators, or successful entrepreneurs. Often, these clients do not regard their therapists as particularly powerful or persuasive but as professional listeners or facilitators (Lazarus & Zur, 2002; Zur, 2005a), and, indeed, they may, simply by virtue of their roles in life, exert a power and influence of their own over the therapist. Regardless of a client's power, the fiduciary relationship is the foundation of the therapist–client relationship and must be preserved at all times by the therapist. Accordingly, a therapist must avoid any interventions that are likely to harm a client, such as a sexual relationship or financial exploitation. Whenever possible, therapists must attempt to minimize potential harm. That is not to say that a therapist who touches a client in a nonsexual manner, accepts an appropriate gift, or crosses boundaries in other ways must anticipate and assure the prevention of all harm, which is not always possible. However, a therapist has a fiduciary obligation to reasonably anticipate foreseeable risks and attempt to avoid, minimize, and manage them (Younggren & Gottlieb, 2004).

In fact, the view of the power differential changes with the angle of the viewer. With the rise of the humanist and feminist movements in the 1960s and 1970s, a different concept of power in therapy was introduced; both humanistic and feminist therapy strove to develop a more authentic and more egalitarian relationship between therapist and client than other therapeutic modalities (Greenspan, 1995). Boundary crossing—primarily self-disclosure, gifts, dual relationships, nonsexual touch, and a variety of out-of-office experiences—is deemed to permit some of the most effective ways to achieve the feminist and humanist goal of authentic and more egalitarian relationships (Williams, 1997).

Although the power differential is valid and real in many psychotherapeutic situations, it is still unfortunate that it has been used, at times, synonymously with exploitation and harm in the ethics literature. Many relationships with a significant differential of power such as parent–child, teacher–student, or coach–athlete, are not inherently exploitative (Tomm, 1993; Zur, 2000). Parental power facilitates children's growth, teachers' authority enables students to learn, and coaches' influence helps athletes to achieve their full, athletic potential. Few, if any, marriage, business, friendship, or therapy relationships are truly equal. Therapists' power, like that of parents, teachers, coaches, politicians, policemen, attorneys, or physicians, can be used or abused. The Hippocratic Oath mandate to "first do no harm" attends exactly to such dangers. The problem of abusive or exploitative power in therapy does not lie within the boundary crossings or dual relationships but emanates from the therapist's propensity to abuse his or her power for selfish gain. Tomm (1993) added, "It is not the power itself that corrupts, it is the disposition to corruption (or lack of personal responsibility) that is amplified by the power" (p. 11).

When dealing with power issues in psychotherapy, it is important to note that therapists' power is not absolute; it also varies. Short-term therapy focusing on symptom reduction or specific, consultative services are less likely to yield a significant power differential compared with long-term or insight-oriented, psychodynamic therapy. Similarly, family or group therapy, behavioral consultation, psychoeducation, and medication consultation are less likely to result in idealization and power differential compared with individual, transference-based therapy. Gonsiorek and Brown (1989) distinguished between therapy in which the transferential relationship plays a primary role and therapy that is short term and offers little opportunity for transferential relationships to develop.

Contrary to the belief that boundary crossing encourages exploitative behavior by therapists, it has been argued that the opportunity for exploitation is proportional to the amount of isolation in a given therapeutic relationship. The absence of boundary crossing and relationships other than those developed in the traditional therapeutic session results in increased isolation. Although privacy is extremely important in psychotherapy, it has to be acknowledged that therapists' power is increased in isolation and when therapists do not disclose because clients tend then to idealize and idolize them. However, dual relationships, self-disclosure, and incidental encounters, when conducted in a professional manner, can all promote a realistic rather than an idealized picture of the therapist. It has been established that most instances of brainwashing and exploitation occur in isolation, including cult experiences and spousal and child abuse (Zur, 2000).

It also takes place in hostage situations in which the victim may even identify with and join cause with the kidnapper. If a client sees her therapist in church every Sunday with his family, for example, she is going to have a more realistic view of him when she sees his wife and his sometimes misbehaving children. Then, when she sees him in the consulting room, and he is no longer an unknown, neutral, or blank-screen therapist, it is doubtful that he will be idealized in an extreme manner. One might argue that sexual exploitation is less likely to occur if the therapist is also working with the client's spouse, friend, and parent or has another community connection with the client, either directly or indirectly through the client's family and friends (Zur, 2005b). Additionally, therapists are less inclined to exploit those with whom they have a long-term or significant relationship outside of therapy. Along the same lines, Tomm (1993) wrote the following:

> Indeed, the additional human connectedness through a dual relationship is far more likely to be affirming, reassuring, and enriching, than exploitative. To discourage all dual relationships in the field is to promote an artificial professional cleavage in the natural *patterns that connect us* as human beings. It is a stance that is far more impoverishing than it is protective. (p. 7)

The confidential therapeutic relationship and the resulting isolation of the therapist–client relationship seems to be a double-edged sword. On one hand, as has been widely acknowledged, it provides the necessary privacy and safety in which clients are more likely to reveal personal or shameful information to their therapists. On the other hand, what has not been widely as acknowledged, it also increases the power differential by increasing the therapist's power. This power can be used or abused (Lazarus & Zur, 2002; Zur, 2000, 2005a).

Slippery Slope and Boundaries

The slippery slope process is described by Gabbard (1994) as "the crossing of one boundary without obvious catastrophic results [making] it easier to cross the next boundary" (p. 284). It refers to the idea that crossing therapeutic boundaries that are seemingly harmless is likely to lead to boundary violations and harm to clients. Similarly, Pope (1990b) stated that "non-sexual dual relationships, while not unethical and harmful per se, foster sexual dual relationships" (p. 688). Some authors have taken the slippery slope idea further. Simon (1991) declared that "The boundary violation precursors of therapist–patient sex can be as psychologically damaging as the actual sexual involvement itself" (p. 614). This argument asserts not only that boundary crossings are likely to result in boundary violations but that the boundary crossings themselves can be as damaging as the potential boundary violations they may lead to. Following a similar line of thought, several other writers describe certain behaviors undertaken by therapists with their clients (e.g., self-disclosure, hugs, home visits, socializing, longer sessions, lunching, exchanging gifts, walks, playing in recreational leagues) that can be precursors to sexual or other violations or the first step on the slippery slope toward harm and exploitation of their clients, sexually or otherwise (Bersoff, 1999; Borys & Pope, 1989; Koocher & Keith-Spiegel, 1998; Lakin, 1991; Rutter, 1989; Sonne, 1994; St. Germaine, 1996; Strasburger, Jorgenson, & Sutherland, 1992).

If one accepts the slippery slope idea, it readily leads to a conclusion such as that of Strasburger et al. (1992), who stated, "Obviously, the best advice to therapists is not to start [down] the slippery slope, and to avoid boundary violations or dual relationships with patients" (pp. 547–548). Similarly, Woody (1988) asserted, "In order to minimize the risk of sexual conduct, policies must prohibit a practitioner from having any contact with the client outside the treatment context and must preclude any type of dual relationships" (p. 188).

The claim that research supports the slippery slope idea is based on statistical findings that almost all harmful boundary violations were preceded by minor boundary crossings (Borys & Pope, 1989; Koocher & Keith-Spiegel, 1998; Lakin, 1991; Rutter, 1989; Sonne, 1994; St. Germaine, 1996; Strasburger et al., 1992). The problem with the statistical argument is that it draws causal conclusions from statistical correlations. As is known from basic research methods and principles, sequential relationships and statistical correlations cannot be equated with causal relationships. Therefore, we cannot say that boundary crossing causes boundary violations just because a boundary crossing happened to precede a boundary violation. Arnold Lazarus (1994), the founder of multimodal therapy and a prominent behavioral therapist, called this slippery slope argument "an extreme form of syllogistic reasoning" (p. 257). Others have argued that to assert that boundary crossings are likely to lead to harm and sex because they statistically precede them is like saying doctors' visits cause death because most people see a doctor before they die (Zur, 2000). The fear that any boundary crossing will result in sexual violations is described by Dineen (1996) as part of the more inclusive problem of the culture at large, including psychotherapists, which is the sexualizing of most boundaries and boundary crossings.

National surveys document that most therapists exchange inexpensive gifts, shake hands, engage in appropriate, nonsexual touch, and almost all self-disclose (e.g., Borys & Pope, 1989; Johnston & Farber, 1996; Pope, Tabachnick, & Keith-Spiegel, 1987). Some of the same surveys (e.g., Pope et al., 1987) also report that between 0.9% and 12.1% of male therapists and between 0.2% and 3% of female therapists have engaged in sexual acts with clients. The discrepancy between the majority of therapists who use boundary crossing to increase effectiveness of treatment and the small minority who commit boundary violations does not lend support to the slippery slope idea that boundary crossings are likely to lead to boundary violations.

On the basis of the logically faulty idea of the slippery slope, an "exploitation index" was developed by Simon and Epstein (Epstein & Simon, 1990; Epstein, Simon, & Kay, 1992). Consistent with Simon's (1994) belief that therapists must "Maintain therapist neutrality. Foster psychological separateness of patient. . . . Ensure no previous, current, or future personal relationships with patients. Minimize physical contact" (p. 514), he and Epstein developed the index listing common and widely practiced boundary crossings such as nonsexual touch, gifts, and dual relationships, in an attempt to identify the variety of boundary crossings and exploitative boundary violations that are likely to be predictors and precursors of therapists' exploitation of their clients.

In this book, I argue that nonsexual therapeutic touch, self-disclosure, small gifts, home visits, and other appropriate boundary crossings can have high clinical utility and a positive effect on the therapeutic alliance and therapeutic outcome. It is important to remember that following the slippery slope rationale and banning or avoiding some appropriate boundary crossings because they may lead to boundary violations may undermine important tenets of humanistic, existential, and feminist-based therapies that emphasize flexibility and embrace boundary crossing, especially self-disclosure. It would also have the effect of reducing the use of cognitive–behavioral and other therapeutic orientations, which regularly incorporate boundary crossing into the treatment plans. Without doubt, it would abolish body psychotherapy that is often based on actual therapeutic touch rather than on verbal exchange. For similar reasons, it would eliminate home visits, case-management-based social work that focuses on home visits, adventure or outdoor therapy, and treating the chronically mentally ill homeless population. It would also deny therapy to those who are cash poor and prefer to barter rather than get free therapy. In a parallel consideration, avoidance of all dual relationships would be impossible in the military, in prisons, and in police departments. Consequently, there could be no psychotherapy services in those systems. Furthermore, it would mean that vast numbers of people living in rural and other small communities would have no access to psychotherapy services.

Transference and Boundaries

The original injunction against any boundary crossing in psychotherapy came from psychoanalytic psychotherapists who were apprehensive about how it would affect the transferential relationships. Any boundary crossing, according to many psychoanalytically oriented therapists, results in contamination of the transference, interference in the analysis of the transference, and the risk of inappropriate self-gratification on the part of the therapist (Johnston & Farber, 1996; Langs, 1982). For that reason, psychoanalysis has issued the injunction against gift exchange, bartering, touch, home visits, or any other boundary crossing. Familiarity that arises from self-disclosure, incidental encounters, or dual relationships has also been seen as compromising the projections necessary for the analysis of transference and countertransference and to the process of securing the consistent and neutral mode of therapy (Epstein & Simon, 1990; Lakin, 1991; Langs, 1982; Lewis, 1959; Simon, 1994).

Transference has emerged as a controversial term in the last couple of decades, especially in the ethics and forensic areas. The debate is about its universality and applicability. On one side of the debate are those who claim that transference is a universal phenomenon that inevitably takes place in and out of the consulting room. As a result, they claim that transference takes place in the consulting room regardless of the therapist's theoretical orientation, method of intervention, or training. In the forensic area, transference has been used to support the claim of clients' inherent vulnerability to therapists' misuse of power. In this view, transference increases therapists' power and, therefore, their ability to exploit their clients. Several courts have supported this stance by accepting the inevitability that transference and countertransference feelings emerge in the course of therapy and the inevitability of clients' vulnerability (Strasburger et al., 1992). Similarly, "transference abuse" was introduced in malpractice litigation and administrative hearings and appears in court rulings synonymously with therapists' misuse of power, exploitation, and boundary violations (Williams, 1997, 2002). On the other side of the debate are those who identify transference in a more limited way and view it principally as a psychoanalytic or psychodynamic construct rather than a universal phenomenon. They view it as a theoretical concept used mainly in psychoanalysis (Lazarus, 1994). Williams (1997) reflected on transference: "because of its overt theoretical linkage to psychoanalysis, causing the concept to be meaningless or offensive to numerous practitioners" (p. 240). Gutheil (1989) pointed out, "It seems that professionals who belong to a school of thought that rejects the idea of transference, behaviorists, or psychiatrists who provide only drug treatment, are being held to a standard of care they do not acknowledge" (p. 31).

Alongside the rising concern about the effect of boundary crossing on transference, a parallel development has taken place in the last couple of decades whereby boundary crossings are used together with transference analysis. As was noted earlier in this book, Freud, Klein, Winnicott, Ferenczi, Jung, and many other early analysts regularly crossed boundaries and physically touched their clients, shared meals with them, took them on vacation, exchanged gifts with them, and loaned money to them while conducting transference analysis as part of the psychoanalytic treatment (Gutheil & Gabbard, 1998; Schoener, 1997; D. Smith & Fitzpatrick, 1995). However, these actions were never incorporated into psychoanalytic theory and instruction in a systematic way. More recently, several authors have discussed the value of integrating boundary crossings such as nonsexual touch (Fosshage, 2000), self-disclosure (Bridges, 2001; Cooper, 1998; Epstein, 1994; Mallow, 1998; Z. D. Peterson, 2002), and gifts (Hahn, 1998) into analytic and transference work. Similarly, Zur (2001a, 2001b) articulated how dual relationships and familiarity do not nullify transference work but only make it more reality, rather than imagination or idealization, based. In any case, regardless of their therapeutic orientation, many therapists are not in a position to use a blank-screen or emotionally neutral type intervention. Those who practice in any kind of small community or on university campuses are known, and often well known, to their clients before, during, and after therapy. Similarly, those who make home visits, work with homeless people on the streets, or conduct adventure therapy are inevitably seen in rather realistic terms.

Although the question about the universality, application, and utility of transference is far from being settled, it is important that clinicians identify their clinical rationale and, when applied, bring theoretical support and ethical reasoning to bear on their decision to use boundary crossing. Similarly, when dual relationships are involved, it is important that therapists identify the communal or other relevant context-related factors of therapy and their ethical reasoning for engaging in dual relationships. Such documentation is likely to protect the clinician from accusations that are based on transference abuse claims. Articulation of therapists' theoretical orientations, used in each intervention, would help establish the fact that they practice within the standard of care as it is defined by the theoretical orientation. As was noted earlier, both the standard of care and the most recent American Psychological Association (2002; see also http://www.apa.org/ethics/) Ethics Code have emphasized the importance of evaluating the appropriateness of therapeutic interventions and therapists' conduct within the context (which includes the theoretical orientation) in which they have taken place, rather than by an arbitrary standard that fits all situations.

3

Contexts of Therapy

It is useful to begin this chapter with an illustration of contexts in therapy. A male therapist takes a resistant but otherwise functional adolescent boy for a walk on a nearby nature trail. In this tranquil and informal ambience, they can talk about the boy's difficulties "side by side" rather than face-to-face. This may be the correct and creative intervention with such a client, particularly in a rural area where young men often feel most comfortable in the outdoors. A high-five might punctuate a successful discussion and the resolution of some of the concerns discussed on the walk. However, the same intervention is likely to be counterindicated, and probably below the standard of care, with an anxious borderline female patient who professes a deep attraction to her therapist. As in this example, this chapter outlines how different clients, different settings, different therapeutic relationships, and, sometimes, different therapists often require different treatment approaches.

The nature, meaning, acceptability, and utility of boundaries in therapy are determined by four factors:

- ☐ *Client factors* include such elements as the client's age, gender, presenting problem, and culture.
- ☐ *Setting of therapy* means the physical location of the sessions (e.g., a hospital, stand-alone clinic, urban or rural locations, etc.).

☐ *Therapy factors* refer to primary theoretical orientation or modality used; type, frequency, and intensity of therapy; and the nature and quality of the therapeutic relationship.

☐ *Therapist factors* include the therapist's age, gender, culture, training, and so on.

Client Factors

Client factors, which include the client's presenting problem, culture, gender, and history, among others, can determine the utility of boundary crossing. For example, whereas a client from a Latino or Middle Eastern culture might be accustomed to—and may initiate—an embrace in greeting, a client of North American or Western European origin may find the handshake to be the most acceptable form of touch when greeting. A home visit, which is appropriate to a bedridden older adult and may be the only way to provide services to this individual, would be highly inappropriate with an able, volatile–impulsive client. Phone or e-mail therapy may be appropriate with a rather high-functioning client but inappropriate with a deeply disturbed, delusional client. Conducting in vivo exposure with a phobic client outside the office may be clinically effective, which is not likely to be the case with a highly paranoid client. Receiving or giving gifts is very common and can be important in child therapy and with clients from Latino, Jewish, and other cultures but not always clinically appropriate with adults who tend to "buy" love and those from cultures in which gift-giving carries heavier symbolic meaning or obligation to reciprocate.

Client factors include the following:

☐ culture, country of origin, acculturation level, and language proficiency;

☐ history, including history of trauma, sexual, or physical abuse;

☐ age;

☐ gender;

☐ presenting problem, mental state, and type and severity of mental disturbances;

☐ socioeconomic class, finances, living conditions, and transportation;

☐ personality type and personality disorders;

☐ sexual orientation;

☐ religious or spiritual beliefs and practices;

☐ social support;

☐ physical health condition and level of physical mobility; and

☐ prior experience with therapy and therapists and general attitudes about mental health care seeking.

Client factors are an exceedingly important consideration when using boundary crossings in therapy whether the boundary crossing is implemented by choice or is unavoidable. Unavoidable boundary crossings such as those likely to occur in many small and rural communities nonetheless require that therapists carefully consider client factors when responding to such occurrences. Treatment plans must be tailored to each client's needs and constructed according to the presenting problem and all other factors previously listed. Ideally, therapists should be so alert to boundaries that they treat boundary crossing with as much consideration as the decision to use a clinical intervention.

Therapeutic Setting

The therapeutic setting component includes issues such as location and type of practice. The following are some important points to remember. A home office environment is much more intimate and self-disclosing than a hospital-based clinic and is obviously not suited for all types of clients or all types of treatments. Conducting therapy on an Indian reservation or on an aircraft carrier does not facilitate anonymity the way a solo private practice in a metropolitan area does. Out-of-office, incidental encounters are common and unavoidable in small college counseling centers and in small towns but are less likely in large urban settings. Bartering for goods may be acceptable in poor, rural, agricultural communities but generally rare in most middle- or upper-class urban areas. Dual relationships are often common and expected in small communities but not as often in major cities. Holding the hand of a dying client for a long time is more expected and appropriate in a hospice-focused or hospital-based practice than in most other therapy settings.

Setting factors include the following:

- ☐ type of practice: outpatient, inpatient, or day programs; solo practice or group practice; freestanding clinic, hospital-based clinic, hospice, or psychiatric emergency unit; privately owned clinic or publicly run agency;
- ☐ locality: large metropolitan area, small rural town, Indian reservation; affluent, suburban setting or poor urban neighborhood; large university counseling center or small college counseling center; major metropolitan setting, remote military base, prison, or police department setting; office in medical building, private setting, or home office;
- ☐ the presence or proximity of a receptionist, staff, other businesses, other professionals, or other psychotherapists;
- ☐ forensic settings and legal mandates: elective therapy, court-mandated evaluation, sanity evaluation, or fitness-for-duty evaluation; hospitalization through voluntary admission or involuntary hold; mandated reporting of abuse of a child, elder, or person or client with mental illness posing imminent danger to self or others; and
- ☐ presence or absence of unavoidable incidental encounters and dual relationships: close community such as deaf, gay male and lesbian, church or other religious group, and ethnic group.

Members of disenfranchised or traditionally oppressed minorities such as the deaf, gay male and lesbian, African American, or certain religious communities, often choose their psychotherapist only after they have gotten to know their values and background and observed them in the community, and thus, most important, developed some trust in them (e.g., Herlihy & Corey, 2006; Kertész, 2002; Kessler & Waehler, 2005; Schank & Skovholt, 2006). What is often required in these situations is boundary crossing in the form of extensive self-disclosure on the part of therapists during the initial phone interview (see chap. 9, this volume). History has taught people who have been oppressed to be suspicious of or at least cautious with members of the mainstream culture and to rely on each other whenever possible. When it comes to psychotherapy, these kinds of populations often prefer a therapist who is one of their own (Liddle, 1997; Sears, 1990) or, at the minimum, familiar with and respectful of their culture. Small and intimate community settings present practitioners with an array of rich and complicated boundary considerations. Incidental encounters are unavoidable and socializing is common and, in fact, expected (e.g., Barnett & Yutrzenka, 1994; Hargrove, 1986; Younggren & Gottlieb, 2004).

Military law imposes complicated mandatory multiple relationships on psychotherapists, and thus military bases provide a clear illustration of how the setting affects a wide array of boundary considerations (Barnett & Yutrzenka, 1994). Needless to say, such complexities radically change the nature of boundaries, including concerns with confidentiality, harm, conflict of interest, and multiple relationships (see chap. 1, this volume).

Therapy Factors

Therapy factors include the quality, intensity, and type of therapeutic relationship or the therapeutic alliance; frequency and length of therapy; people involved in therapy; and therapeutic orientation used. For example, self-disclosure varies significantly between therapeutic orientations. Whereas some self-disclosure is almost always embedded in humanistic or feminist psychotherapy, it is clinically contraindicated for traditional, transference-based psychoanalytic psychotherapy. Posttherapy social dual relationships between clients and therapists are more likely to be less problematic in short-term and psychoeducational therapies than in long-term psychodynamic therapy.

Therapy factors encompass both therapeutic factors and therapeutic relationship factors. Therapeutic factors include the following:

- □ modality: individual, couple, family, or group therapy; short term, long term, or intermittent long-term therapy;

- intensity–frequency: therapy sessions several times a week or once-a-month consultation;
- population: child, adolescent, or adult psychotherapy; and
- theoretical orientation: psychoanalysis, humanistic, group therapy, body psychotherapy, eclectic therapy.

Therapeutic relationship factors include the following:

- quality and nature of therapeutic alliance: secure, trusting, tentative, fearful, or safe connection; intense and involved, neutral, or casual relationships;
- length: new or long-term relationship;
- period: beginning of therapy, middle of therapy, or toward termination;
- idealized–transferential relationships or familiar and more egalitarian relationships;
- mutual respect, liking, and trust or mutual disrespect (contempt), dislike, fear, and distrust;
- familiarity and interactivity in the community or only-in-the-office, circumscribed relationship; and
- presence or absence of dual relationships and type of dual relationships, if applicable.

Theoretical orientations espoused by therapists are likely to be among the most significant factors determining a therapist's approach to boundaries (Borys & Pope, 1989; Gutheil & Gabbard, 1993, 1998; Lazarus & Zur, 2002; Williams, 1997). Family therapists are likely to define the boundaries of psychotherapy, including the limits of confidentiality and who is a patient, in a broader way than most individual therapists (Minuchin, 1974).

Psychoanalytically oriented therapists, for clinical reasons, are likely to avoid physical touch and gifts, to remain emotionally neutral, and to set a clear and consistent start and finish to the therapeutic hour (Langs, 1982; Simon, 1991). At the other end of the spectrum, a humanistic therapist is likely to be more flexible with regard to physical touch, exchange of gifts, and beginning and end of sessions. He or she may even leave the office with a client for an out-of-office session (Jourard, 1971b; Zur, 2001b). A behavioral therapist may choose to leave the office as part of a systematic desensitization of a client with a specific phobia (Gutheil & Gabbard, 1993; Lazarus, 1994). Another prime example is self-disclosure. A feminist therapist may make a point of inviting or joining a client for a political rally to manifest the ideology of breaking down boundaries and to emphasize the importance of political involvement (Greenspan, 1986; Hanson, 2003). Similarly, humanistic therapists emphasize the importance of self-disclosure for the forming of authentic therapist–patient relationships (Bugental, 1987; Jourard, 1971a), and cognitive–behavioral therapists may reveal personal information for the purpose of modeling (Dryden, 1990; Lazarus, 1998). Obviously, a body psychotherapist, such as a Reichian or bioenergetic practitioner, will extensively use touch rather than words in the course of psychotherapy (Reich, 1972). A family or behavioral therapist may choose to join an anorexic client for a family dinner as part of the treatment plan (Fay, 2002; Minuchin, 1974). The spiritually oriented or pastoral counselor often joins a client in prayer and at services (Llewellyn, 2002). It is thus apparent that therapists' primary theoretical orientations determine their view of what constitutes appropriate and helpful practice with regard to boundaries in psychotherapy.

To illustrate the differences between orientations, I have included the following often-cited quotes by analytic and humanistic scholars, representing the range of opinion regarding therapeutic boundaries. Simon (1994), who has often been the voice of the traditional analytic stance on boundaries, stated the following:

> Maintain therapist neutrality. Foster psychological separateness of the patient. Obtain informed consent for treatment and procedures. Interact verbally with clients. Ensure no previous, current, or future personal relationships with patients. Minimize physical contact. Preserve relative anonymity of the therapist. Establish a stable fee policy. Provide a consistent, private, and professional setting. Define length and time of sessions. (p. 514)

Jourard (1971b), who often has been considered to represent the humanistic psychology point of view on boundaries, stated the following:

> In the context of dialogue, I don't hesitate to share any of my experience with existential binds roughly comparable to those

in which the seeker finds himself (this is now called "modeling"); nor do I hesitate to disclose my experience of him, myself, and our relationship as it unfolds from moment to moment. . . . I might give Freudian or other types of interpretations. I might teach him such Yoga know-how or tricks for expanding body-awareness as I have mastered or engage in arm wrestling or hold hands or hug him, if that is the response that emerges in the dialogue. (p. 159)

Research on the relationships between therapists' orientations and practices has yielded several results. Pope, Tabachnick, and Keith-Spiegel's (1987) and Borys and Pope's (1989) extensive surveys revealed that boundary crossing such as self-disclosure, small gift-giving, and nonsexual touching was surprisingly prevalent in the practices of psychologists and other psychotherapists across all theoretical orientations. Borys and Pope's findings support the claim that maintenance of boundaries is related to therapeutic orientation especially among psychodynamic and humanistic practitioners. A study of "everyday" boundaries in psychotherapy such as ending sessions on time, requiring timely payment of fees, and demanding adherence to specified appointment times, reveals that most therapists, regardless of their theoretical orientation, report that they are flexible and work cooperatively with clients on these issues (Johnston & Farber, 1996). However, it should be noted that "humanistic" was not one of the choices for assigning theoretical orientation in this study.

Therapist Factors

Therapist factors include gender, age, culture, and sexual orientation. They also include scope and type of training, that is, education, internships, supervision, and postgraduate education and consultations. For example, a young and attractive woman therapist must be more cautious in using physical touch or leaving the office when working with a heterosexual male client than would a male therapist of any age.

Similar to client factors, therapist factors are closely tied to age, culture, gender, and sexual orientation. Interventions that are likely to be appropriate if implemented by a male therapist may be inappropriate for a female therapist. Similarly, a young therapist may use gestures, language, and mannerisms that are age specific or age appropriate. An older therapist, using the same language or mannerisms, may appear inauthentic and may harm the therapeutic alliance. A therapist trained in body psychotherapy and somatic therapies is more likely to use touch in the course of psychotherapy than a psychodynamically trained therapist and most other therapists.

A therapist's culture is obviously another significant factor in the therapeutic consideration of boundaries. A Native American therapist would much more naturally join a ritual with a local shaman if it is clinically appropriate than a non–Native American therapist, just as a Jewish therapist would feel at ease attending a ritual circumcision (*bris*) or other Jewish ritual.

A therapist's training and professional socialization are also highly relevant to the way he or she is likely to treat boundaries. Therapists who were trained in case management and conducted regular home visits or those whose internship was with the homeless are more likely to consider leaving the office for clinical reasons than those who were never trained in such clinical interventions.

A generation gap among therapists, reflected in attitudes and practices around boundary issues, has been observed in recent years. Psychotherapists who were trained in fairly recent years may tend to adhere more closely to conservative boundary guidelines than those trained in prior decades. A national survey by Borys and Pope (1989) found a significant relationship between therapists' years of experience and their ratings concerning the ethics of maintaining dual professional roles with patients, with less experienced therapists more likely to consider dual roles unethical. The reasons for such shifts may lie in changes in graduate and professional education or in the more recent proliferation of risk management practices (Williams, 1997). The implications of this generation gap are still not clear. Possibly, younger therapists' more conservative views of ethical practices in general and of boundaries in particular may translate to a more restrictive standard of care. One may also wonder, with the shift in the American Counseling Association (2005, see also http://www.

counseling.org/Resources/CodeOfEthics/TP/Home/CT2.aspx), the American Psychological Association (2002; see also http://www.apa.org/ethics/) Ethics Code, and in professional literature toward more flexible and context-based therapeutic boundaries, including dual relationships, if the generation gap may one day narrow or even disappear.

Obviously, therapists' history and experience are relevant to their capacity to use self-disclosure. Clients commonly establish trusting and positive therapeutic relationships with therapists whose own life experiences parallel those of the client such as experiences in war, with addiction, as a parent as well as a similar religious or spiritual orientation, sexual orientation, or ethnic background (Barnett, 1998; Geyer, 1994; M. Jones, Botsko, & Gorman, 2003; Llewellyn, 2002; Sears, 1990).

The meaning of therapeutic boundaries and the utility of boundary crossings can only be comprehended within the context of therapy. This context is composed of four factors: client, setting, therapy, and therapist. Although the basic protection of the confidential relationship, welfare of clients, and injunction against sexual dual relationships and other exploitative relationships are almost always constant across settings, cultures, theoretical orientations, and therapists, the meaning of boundaries varies significantly from context to context. What may be appropriate and useful in one context may be inappropriate and harmful in another. When evaluating the meaning of a boundary to the clients and to therapy, those basic four factors must be carefully considered.

4

A Decision-Making Process for Boundary Crossing and Dual Relationships

This chapter briefly reviews the literature on general ethical decision making, decision making vis-à-vis dual relationships, and basic principles of critical thinking and risk–benefit analysis. It then provides a seven-step process for ethical decision making with regard to boundary crossing.

Ethical Decision Making

Ethical decision making in psychotherapy has received much attention. Many texts have focused on the principles of ethics in psychology (e.g., Beauchamp & Childress, 2001; Kitchener, 1988). As with the general principles of the American Psychological Association (2002; see also http://www.apa.org/ethics/) Ethics Code, they view the following five moral principles as the foundation of ethical decision making: (a) *autonomy,* the concept whereby the clients' freedom of choice is respected and encouraged and the responsibility for actions and how they affect the self and others is stressed; (b) *nonmaleficence,* the principle of "do no harm," which involves not intentionally inflicting pain on others and refraining from actions that risk harm to others; (c) *beneficence,* the counselor's responsibility to contribute to the client's well-being by preventing harm and being proactive in attempting to benefit the client; (d) *justice,* the principle of providing equal treatment for all clients; and (e) *fidelity*, honoring commitments and guarding the client's trust and the therapeutic relationship.

Several texts outline ethical decision making for psychotherapists as being broad and inclusive and, as such, cover general ethical decision making as well as concerns with therapeutic boundaries (e.g., Canter, Bennett, Jones, & Nagy, 1996; Corey, Corey, & Callahan, 2003; Haas & Malouf, 1989; Herlihy & Corey, 2006; Knapp & VandeCreek, 2006; Koocher & Keith-Spiegel, 1998; Welfel, 2002). Most of the ethical decision-making models identify several basic steps that constitute the ethical decision-making process. These steps include the following: identifying the relevant ethical conflicts involved; identifying the relevant section of the professional code of ethics; developing alternative courses of action; conducting a risk–benefit analysis of the likely short- and long-term consequences of each course of action on the individual or group involved or likely to be affected; making an informed choice of course of action applying the relevant ethical principles; evaluating the results of the course of action; and modifying the course of action as required or reengaging in the decision-making process, if necessary. Most of the models also emphasize the importance of involving the client in different junctions of the process.

Ethical Decision Making Regarding Boundary Crossings and Dual Relationships

A few texts focus on ethical decision making and guidelines with regard to boundary crossings and dual relationships. Koocher and Keith-Spiegel (1998), Gutheil and Gabbard (1993), Corey et al. (2003), Herlihy and Corey (2006), Knapp and VandeCreek (2006), Reamer (2001), Schank and Skovholt (2006), D. Smith and Fitzpatrick (1995), and Welfel (2002), among others, provided guidelines for handling boundary crossing in therapy. Some others have provided more specific guidelines such as those for handling nonsexual touch (Hunter & Struve, 1998; Nordmarken & Zur, 2004; E. Smith, Chance, & Imes, 1998), gifts (Knox, Hess, Williams, & Hill, 2003; Smolar, 2003), bartering (Hill, 1999), or self-disclosure (Barnett, 1998; Z. D. Peterson, 2002).

Several other authors have provided more specific models and guidelines for handling dual relationship situations. Kitchener (1988) based her model on role theory and centered on the role conflicts created in dual relationships. Her model listed three guidelines to differentiate between dual relationships that are likely to be problematic and those that are less likely to lead to conflicts. The first guideline concerned incompatibility of role expectations such as between the clinical and the social. The second guideline stated that as the obligations of different roles diverge, the potential for divided loyalties and loss of objectivity increases. The third guideline stated that as the power and prestige differential between client and therapist increases, so does the potential for exploitation. On the basis of this role theory model, in part, S. K. Anderson and Kitchener (1998) proposed an ethical decision-making model for posttherapy nonsexual dual relationships. They identified eight different dual relationships in which psychologists may engage. These relationships vary from incidental and unavoidable to intentional relationships formed after the therapeutic contact. Their model presented a series of questions around the following four general concerns in deciding to enter a posttherapy relationship: the initial therapeutic contract and termination considerations; the dynamics and strength of the therapeutic bond, power differential, and potential of the new relationship to be counterclinical; the social role and expectations; and the therapist's motivation for seeking or having a dual relationship.

Gottlieb's (1993) model used three dimensions to assess the potential for harm from dual relationships: power differential, duration of treatment, and termination and potential future clinical engagements. Gottlieb suggested that the psychologist assess the current relationship, its nature, and intensity and evaluate the role incompatibility of the dual relationship and possible role conflict. Ebert (1997) provided a comprehensive model for ethical decision making for dual relationships that is based on conflict of interest. He argued that the construct of dual relationships is not very useful because dual relationships can be unavoidable and helpful. Hence, it is not the dual relationship per se but its potential to harm through conflict of interest that can lead to ethical violations. Lazarus and Zur (2002) provided a simpler decision-making model, which is based on clients' specific needs, the setting, and above all whether the dual relationships are likely to be harmful, helpful, or inconsequential. Finally, Younggren and Gottlieb (2004) suggested the following five questions for therapists who attempt to manage risk associated with dual relationships: (a) Is entering into a relationship in addition to the professional one necessary, or should I avoid it? (b) Can the dual relationship potentially cause harm to the client? (c) If harm seems unlikely or avoidable, would the additional relationship prove beneficial? (d) Is there a risk that the dual relationship could disrupt the therapeutic relationship? (e) Can I evaluate this matter objectively?

In addition to these specific models for ethical decision making regarding dual relationships, several other articles incorporated a decision-making process into their discussion of dual relationships (e.g., Barnett, 1999; Gutheil & Gabbard, 1993; Herlihy & Corey, 2006; Koocher & Keith-Spiegel, 1998; Sterling, 1992). These texts acknowledge that dual relationships are not always avoidable, focus on the code of ethics, and stress the importance of context issues such as the type and length of therapy and setting or communal considerations. Additionally, they all underscore the importance of awareness of potential conflict of interest.

Risk–Benefit Analysis of Action and Inaction

Therapists should ask themselves certain questions before deciding to cross a boundary. The same is true before deciding whether it is ethical to make a home visit or accept a gift. In the spirit of critical thinking, therapists must consider which questions are the right ones to ask.

These questions may be, "Should I cross this boundary (e.g., should I accept this gift)?" "Is it ethical to cross this boundary (i.e., is it ethical to accept this particular gift)?" or "What are the risks and benefits of carrying out or not carrying out the proposed action (i.e., what are the potential risks and benefits of either accepting or rejecting the gift)?" Questions, such as the first two, that focus on whether to cross or not to cross a certain boundary or whether a certain action is ethical or not, are likely to generate a narrower analysis than the latter question that focuses on the risks and benefits of doing or not doing something. The question "Should I accept this gift?" is likely to be met with a response such as, "Yes, accepting this gift is likely to enhance the client's sense of self and strengthen the relationship between me and my client who is struggling with low self-esteem and her relationship with rejecting parents" or "No, accepting this gift is likely to support the client's belief that she can be loved only if she gives gifts." Responding to the question, "Is it ethical to accept the gift?" may be answered by "Yes, it is ethical to accept this small symbolic gift as it does not pose any risk of exploitation, does not raise a concern with conflict of interest or loss of objectivity, and, therefore, nothing in the codes of ethics would indicate that it is unethical." Responding to the risk–benefit question invites a broader analysis that includes both potential harm and potential benefit for following or not following the course of action. For example, the risk of accepting a gift from this particular client involves affirming her belief that she is not lovable, interferes with the transference analysis, and may give her the impression that the therapist is greedy. However, accepting the gift is likely to enhance the therapeutic alliance and allow the client to experience the therapist's expression of gratitude. The risk of not accepting the gift is that the client may experience shame, rejection, and an irrevocable rupture of the therapeutic alliance, especially if the client's cultural background is such that refusing a gift is likely to be perceived as an insult. Rejection of the gift may result in the client dropping out of therapy. The potential benefit of not accepting the gift is that it may enable the client to become conscious of and verbally articulate her desire to be accepted and loved rather than "acting it out" by buying love through gift giving.

Decision-making processes that are solely based on "do no harm" without including the balancing mandate to act in the client's best interest are inherently defective and are likely to yield flawed conclusions. Therapists cannot make the unilateral decision to "do no harm." Such an attempt may eliminate some of the most promising clinical interventions and therapeutic modalities. The ethical imperative is to act competently and in the best interest of clients and not to exploit them. With rare exceptions, such as sexual relationships and other blatant, exploitative actions, a rational recommendation cannot be made about the ethical status of an action without knowing both its potential risks and the potential benefits.

Risk–benefit analysis of actions or inactions brings to the forefront the contexts of therapy (i.e., client factors, setting, therapy, and therapist factors; see chap. 3, this volume), which must be included in any analysis, and the fact that all clinical interventions, regardless of how well thought out and well meaning they are, also contain risk. As a matter of fact, any human action and any human inaction are associated with some level of risk.

Additional rarely discussed concerns are actual physical risks to therapists and their families. Working with violent, volatile, threatening, or vindictive clients may pose such threats to therapists. Similarly, clients who follow or stalk their therapists or their families also pose a risk. Working from one's home, conducting home visits, using adventure therapy, and other interventions outside the traditional office may also be associated with higher risk to the therapist. When relevant, these types of considerations should enter into the risk–benefit analysis.

Risk management has been one of the major concerns when making decisions regarding boundaries. As a result, the question "Should I accept (or give) this gift?" is often answered negatively because of the risks posed by possible confrontation with boards and ethics committees or because it may be perceived negatively in court. (The concern with the negative effects of risk management, or what has been called "practicing defensive medicine," on the quality and integrity of care is described in more detail in the Introduction.) However, if the question is articulated more broadly and includes risk–benefit analysis for action and inaction, risk management considerations are only one component that should be weighed against many other factors, primarily those involving the best interests of the client. Therefore, risk–benefit analyses do not simply reject boundary crossing because it involves risk, instead they invite therapists to ask the question, "Do these risks outweigh the benefits?" or "Are these risks justified?" Therapists must take into consideration that they can actually *do* harm through inaction and in the attempt to avoid harm (Fay, 2002; Lazarus & Zur, 2002). Of course, therapists must be committed to preventing and deterring intentional harm and negligent harm. Risk–benefit analysis also eliminates taking unnecessary risks.

The following is an example of a clinical record detailing briefly a risk–benefit analysis:

> Accepting the handmade scarf from a client was weighed against rejecting it. While accepting it might reinforce the client's belief that she needs to give in order to be loved, rejecting it would be a reenactment of her parents' rejection of her. Rather than a blanket acceptance or rejection of the gift, it was placed aside, next to the client and the therapist, while they engaged in a discussion of its meaning. The client was able to understand the complexity and dual nature of her gift-giving and gained awareness of both her attempt to express gratitude and her impulse to buy love. Once such understanding about the meaning and the intent of the gift-giving was achieved, the gift was accepted.

A Decision-Making Process

This section presents a seven-step decision-making process that uses the codes of ethics to augment critical thinking and to emphasize flexibility and clinical effectiveness. As it takes a broad approach to the decision-making process, important concerns such as power differential, length and intensity of the therapeutic relationship, and transference, are incorporated into the proposed model and are attended to when necessary and applicable. Partly on the basis of the previously mentioned ethical decision-making models and incorporating moral and critical-thinking principles, among others, the following is the progression for ethical decision making for boundaries in psychotherapy.

The first step is identifying the issue. This can vary from the suitability of accepting a gift, to consulting with a certain client at the therapist's home office, to the propriety of establishing a bartering relationship, to the suitability of dual relationships that will result from accepting a fellow congregation member as a client.

The second step is identifying the relevant moral, ethical, clinical, legal, professional, communal, and other issues and conflicts involved. These may include concern with the client's welfare, the client's family, and the client's community, or possibly the hospital or military institution where the client is located. Issues of nonmaleficence, beneficence, fidelity, responsibility, justice, respect, and integrity are all of great consequence to this step. The codes of ethics are especially pertinent to this stage, but the inquiry may include additional moral, philosophical, spiritual, and community values, as well as other germane considerations. The entire context of therapy, which includes client, setting, therapy, and therapist factors, should be considered at this early stage of the decision-making process (see chap. 3, this volume). At this point, some conflicting issues may arise. Making a home visit or attending a wedding may be clinically advised but may compromise the client's privacy and confidentiality, may pose physical danger to the clinician, may be viewed as risky by risk management experts, and may be disallowed by the clinic or the institution where therapy takes place. If a client offers the therapist a gift, the clinical, moral, cultural, spiritual, economical, and relational aspects of the gift may be relevant even if they may be in conflict with each other. Entering into dual relationships with a client may be appropriate for the client from a clinical point of view but may affect other members in the community negatively.

This stage is aimed at brainstorming or mapping, as broadly as possible, the ethical, professional, and other relevant complexities, not resolving them. Prematurely narrowing the scope of the questioning and inquiry because of risk management or any other concerns risks ruling out potentially valid options and may lead to an unsubstantiated, unethical, or even harmful decision. When trying to identify the ethical issues involved, one may realize that the concerns are not always ethical but some are purely clinical or legal. Involving a consultant may help broaden the possibilities that are considered, and involving the client at this brainstorming stage may be helpful, too, depending on the client and other factors. Question each element, allowing the imagination a free rein but testing each thought critically against all the values that are the best part of the profession of psychotherapy.

The third step is to develop a series of alternative courses of action. Like the second step, this step invites the therapist to think broadly and consider as many options as possible. Reducing the options prematurely may distort the process and create an undesirable course of action. Although risk management concerns should be considered when they are appropriate, it is imperative that they should not interfere with the development of alternative courses of action. Even though many scholars have warned that boundary crossing should be avoided because of the risks to therapists, all options that could benefit the client should nevertheless be considered during this phase. Concerns with the physical safety of clients, therapists, or others should also be included in the development of courses of actions.

The fourth step is conducting an analysis of the likely short-term, ongoing, and long-term risks and benefits of each course of action or inaction for anyone or anything involved or likely to be affected. Besides the individual client, this may include the client's family, loved ones, employees, place of employment, the therapist, colleagues, community, or society. Such evaluations of pros and cons of certain actions and the avoidance of these actions can be highly complicated and difficult. The pros and the cons must take into consideration clinical, ethical, and legal aspects, as well as the standard of care. This leads to a consideration of the contexts of therapy (see chap. 3, this volume). This step can present contradictory options and even opposing courses of actions. As in the second step, involving an expert consultant and engaging the client may be useful.

The fifth step involves first separately weighing the risks against the benefits within each option, then comparing them and choosing a course of action. The chosen course of action will rarely be ideal or perfect; it is only what seems best under the carefully examined circumstances. This course of action is likely to best fit the unique context of therapy that is under consideration. Therapists facing complex ethical, clinical, or legal cases would assuredly benefit from consultation with appropriate experts. There are several ways for therapists to find suitable expert–consultants. Graduate or postgraduate instructors, experienced supervisors, widely published authors, or reputable attorneys can provide expert advice. So can expert–consultants who are recommended by national or state professional associations or a therapist's malpractice insurance company. When seeking a consultant, a therapist must be able to differentiate between ethical, clinical, legal, and risk management types of advice. It is important that a thera-pist is aware, preferably prior to the consultation, of the orienta-tions, biases, and attitudes of the consultant. Because opinions about boundaries are wildly diverse and often contradictory, seek-ing a second or even third opinion from experts of diverse opin-ions will help a therapist make an informed decision.

Therapists must remember that applying such a thorough pro-cess (and documenting it) aligns them with the standard of care. Therapists are not judged by the outcome of their actions, as there is no guarantee that there will be no harm. They are judged by the integrity of their methodologies and decision-making processes. For example, the fact that a client committed suicide is not, by itself, an indication that the therapist was negligent or operated below the standard of care. What determines whether the thera-pist was negligent are his or her decision-making process and actions prior to the death and whether he or she conducted a thor-ough suicide risk assessment, considered voluntary or involun-tary hospitalizations, assessed for availability of firearms, used a crisis intervention modality, and so on. Therapists are evaluated and judged by the rationale for the interventions and process embedded in the decision-making process, and finally by their actions or lack of actions.

The following is an example of a therapist who meticulously followed the proper process, which nonetheless had an undesir-able outcome:

> A middle-aged, male client requested that his therapist make a home visit to enable the therapist to see his home remodel-ing project, of which he was very proud, and at the same time to visit with his dying grandmother. The therapist had spent many sessions discussing the many potential issues attend-ing such a visit. She explored whether the client had sexual or other fantasies about her and the visit, as well as his idea of introducing her to his grandmother or to other people who might come to the house at the time of the proposed visit. She covered privacy and confidentiality issues, the exact location and safety of the neighborhood, the payment consideration associated with such a visit, and many more issues. Addition-ally, the therapist hired an expert consultant to discuss the

ethical and clinical issues involved in this visit, as well as to conduct a thorough risk–benefit analysis. Three months later, the therapist visited the house. The visit turned out to be very negative from a clinical point of view. The client was disappointed with what he perceived to be the short time the therapist allocated to the visit and her lack of interest in his grandmother and in his project. He quit therapy immediately thereafter. This case demonstrates that even though the clinical outcome was negative, the therapist clearly acted within the standard of care as was documented in her comprehensive decision-making process and consultations.

The sixth step involves implementing the course of action chosen through the risk–benefit analysis. This involves articulating a treatment plan, which includes short-term and, when necessary, intermediate and long-term goals; using interventions with the aim of achieving these goals; outlining a theoretical–clinical rationale or empirical support for the proposed interventions; and establishing ways to evaluate the effectiveness of the interventions. The following is a brief example of a treatment plan that involved leaving the office, a clear boundary crossing:

> The goal of the therapy with John, a middle-aged, successful businessman who had no history of mental treatment, and who recently developed agoraphobia, was to diminish his avoidance of open spaces. An in vivo desensitization program was presented, discussed with the client, and implemented with his consent. The discussion included potential concern with privacy and confidentiality that might arise while being outside the office. After doing imaginal desensitization in the office, the next step of the program was the in vivo exposure where therapist and client left the office and went to a nearby open space and took progressively longer walks together.

The seventh step involves developing ways to assess the success or effectiveness of the plan and respond to the results of the assessment by either continuing with it if it has proved successful or modifying or discontinuing it if it has failed to accomplish some or all of its objectives. In the latter case, the therapist should reengage in the decision-making procedure and develop an alternative course of action and a modified or new treatment plan.

In summary, this chapter outlines the basic steps of general ethical decision making that therapists must take before engaging in boundary crossings and dual relationships with clients. It invites the reader to go the length of the decision-making process and to include critical thinking, taking into consideration that all interventions and all inaction involve risk. A thorough risk–benefit analysis of each boundary crossing should be complemented with a risk–benefit analysis of not crossing the specific boundary. The chapter emphasizes that risk management is only one consideration among many others and cautions against placing risk management above clinical considerations. Only by understanding the risk of inaction can therapists make informed decisions about their interventions. Ultimately, the chapter argues, risk management and a thorough decision-making process are not mutually exclusive if there are good clinical records, which include a summary of the decision-making process, the treatment plan, and a review of any consultations.

II

Boundaries Around the Therapeutic Encounter

Time and Money: Managing Time, Fees, Billing, and Bartering

Time and money are two of the most important elements forming the therapeutic frame. They delineate the time borders of
therapy, identify it as a form of business or fee-for-service relationship, and differentiate it from social and other relationships.
For that reason it is important to establish the time and length of
session and fee schedule as early as possible in therapy and preferably, if possible, before it even starts. Although both time and money
agreements may need to be reevaluated and renegotiated during
the course of therapy, they must, in any case, be agreed on initially
and be clearly established each time the agreement is revised.

Time

Time is a primary boundary in psychotherapy because it defines
the beginning and end of sessions and provides a fundamental
frame around the therapeutic encounter. Time is also important
when therapeutic encounters take place outside the office walls.
These situations may involve emergency phone calls, between-
session e-mails, or sessions that are conducted in person outside
the office via phone, e-mail, or videoconferencing. The boundary
marked by time and duration of sessions provides a structure and
containment for clients and therapists alike.

Some of the most frequently discussed time issues have revolved around the beginning and end of sessions, sessions that are longer than planned, unusually lengthy scheduled sessions, sessions scheduled at odd or very late hours, and the scheduling of particular clients for the last session of the day. Like any boundary crossing, it is of utmost importance that any variation from common practices will be carried out with the client's welfare in mind. Allowing a session to run significantly over the allotted time for a client who is clearly in crisis and in need of immediate assistance can be an ethically and clinically appropriate boundary crossing. So is a midnight phone session with an acutely suicidal client. Scheduling a teacher, a nurse, or factory worker for sessions after work or late in the day because the client cannot attend sessions during regular, daytime working hours is appropriate and understandable. Similarly, flexibility in scheduling extra sessions at a client's request and when it is clinically indicated is likely to enhance the therapeutic alliance and clinical outcome (Johnston & Farber, 1996). In contrast, deliberately scheduling clients at the end of the day for personal rather than clinical reasons—such as mutual attraction—when no other clients are arriving for sessions or no staff or other therapists are present is clinically and ethically inappropriate and may constitute a boundary violation. Such late scheduling has been a frequently cited risk management concern (Gabbard & Nadelson, 1995; Gutheil & Gabbard, 1993; Strasburger, Jorgenson, & Sutherland, 1992).

Psychotherapists have been reported to be rather flexible about start of therapy, with nearly 40% of sessions beginning earlier or later than the scheduled time. However, the length of sessions seemed to be much more strictly enforced, with almost all therapists keeping the session to its fully scheduled length or going a few minutes over regardless of the starting time (Johnston & Farber, 1996). Although punctuality does not seem to be a major concern of most therapists, several analytically oriented authors have emphasized the importance of promptness to the analytic process and to clients with chaotic backgrounds (Epstein, 1994; Gutheil & Gabbard, 1993; Simon, 1994).

MediCal, Medicare, and insurance companies have raised additional concerns related to time in recent years. Their concern has been that psychotherapists in general, and psychiatrists conducting medication evaluation in particular, spend less actual time with clients than reported on their invoices. As a result, the Health Insurance Portability and Accountability Act regulations have developed a new mandate for therapists to report beginning and ending time of sessions in the medical records (Zur, 2005b).

Time, as with any other boundary in therapy, can be maintained, crossed, or violated by clients as well as therapists. Time boundaries are crossed when a client is reluctant to leave a session, enters or bursts into the consulting room outside the hour of the appointment, or follows or stalks the therapist outside the office. Some clients demand extra sessions before their therapists go on vacation, insist on phone or e-mail sessions in between sessions, or insist on extra, personal contact when therapists are out of town. The most popular satiric manifestation of such demands on a therapist's time, in this case during the therapist's vacation, is in the movie *What About Bob?* Bill Murray plays an obsessive–compulsive and regressed client who cannot separate from his psychiatrist, played by Richard Dreyfuss, and follows his distressed psychiatrist on his family vacation (Oz, Sargent, Ziskin, & Schulman, 1991). Separating during vacation time is a concern that is experienced not only by clients but also by therapists. Freud analyzed Ferenczi while walking through the countryside during his vacation and Melanie Klein analyzed Clifford Scott for 2 hours every day in her hotel room (Gutheil & Gabbard, 1993).

Interrupted sessions or interference with scheduled therapeutic times constitutes crossing of the boundary of the therapy time frame. This may involve therapists or clients using their cell phones or therapists answering their office phone during sessions. It also includes therapists answering the door or communicating with the secretary or staff on matters not directly related to the client during session time. Multitasking during phone or other telehealth therapy sessions can also interfere with the sanctioned therapeutic time. As technology continues to proliferate and communication devices become more portable, user friendly, and popular, intrusions of such devices into the therapeutic hours seem inevitable. As cell phone use continues to spill over into other activities such as driving, standing in checkout lines, and attending classes or the theater, the therapeutic connection is no longer immune from intrusion by various communication devices.

Telehealth or e-therapy introduces additional complexities with regard to time of therapy. Synchronous communications such as Instant Messaging, chat rooms, videoconferencing, or audioconferencing can have a beginning and end time and are rather similar to in-office, in-person therapy. However, when it comes to asynchronous communication such as e-mail-based therapy, it is hard to determine when and for how long direct and indirect therapy services actually take place (see chap. 8, this volume, for more details).

Fees, Billing, and Other Money Concerns

Like time, the therapist's fee is another basic parameter that defines the therapeutic relationship, differentiating it from social, romantic, or other nonprofessional relationships. Money is the most obvious boundary that defines the business aspect of therapeutic relationships (Gutheil & Gabbard, 1993). The concerns with regard to fees have evolved primarily around issues of sliding scale, no-fee arrangements, bartering, and client nonpayment resulting in client indebtedness. Additional concerns may involve third-party billing, payment for missed or canceled appointments, and fee splitting. Loans and gifts to clients by therapists or to therapists by clients and financial or business dual relationships are discussed in chapter 1.

Many clients cannot afford the therapist's full fee. Correspondingly, psychologists and all others in the helping profession have an ethical commitment to serve those populations that cannot afford to pay the full fee. The American Psychological Association (APA, 2002) Ethics Code, Principle D: Justice, states: "Psychologists recognize that fairness and justice entitle all persons to access and benefit from the contributions of psychology and to equal quality in the processes, procedures, and services being conducted by psychologists" (p. 1062). Most other professional organizations' codes contain a similar commitment. Accordingly, most therapists offer a sliding scale, low-fee, or no-fee arrangement to clients who cannot afford their full or reduced fee. Alternative fee schedules to full-fee, third-party payment or alternative payment methods (e.g., bartering, discussed later in this chapter), sliding scale, or low or no fee have fallen into the category of boundary crossing because they cross the standard, full-fee schedule arrangement boundary (Gutheil & Gabbard, 1993). At the beginning of therapy, therapists and clients must be clear about the fee schedule and how late payments are handled (Koocher & Keith-Spiegel, 1998). Because of changes in economic status or insurance coverage or for emotional reasons, some clients fall behind in their payments. Not collecting fees in a timely manner and allowing a client's debt to accumulate have been frequently cited as clinical or ethical boundary concerns. The primary concern is that if a client's debt grows without the therapist openly discussing the problem, negotiating and revising the original fee agreement, or agreeing on a new payment schedule, it can negatively affect the clinical process. Negotiating a new fee or payment schedule must not only be discussed and agreed on with clients but also be documented in the treatment records. Similarly, forgiving a client's debt should be handled with clinical sensitivity, and its rationale should be documented in the treatment records.

Contracting a collection agency to collect unpaid debts is a clear boundary crossing, because therapists who contact such agencies cross the therapeutic boundary and introduce or involve a third party. The original fee discussion should indicate that clients must be notified beforehand that a collection agency may be notified if they do not pay their bills. Therapists have been strongly advised to try to come to a mutually satisfactory agreement with clients before contacting a collection agency. Prior to the risk management era, one study found that 61% of professional psychologists surveyed used a collection agency (Faustman, 1982). Risk management experts accurately warn that involving a collection agency may lead to a licensing board complaint by the client and, therefore, they strongly advise against it (Bennett, Bryant, VandenBos, & Greenwood, 1990; Woody, 1988).

Therapists loaning money to clients, clients loaning money to therapists, or financial gifts (beyond a dollar for the bus) by either one are additional, challenging boundary issues as they involve additional business or financial dual relationships between therapists and clients. As was discussed in chapter 1 of this volume, such secondary relationships can be highly complicated because they can lead to a conflict-of-interest situation and interfere with the clinical process.

Fee splitting, or what is better known as a *kickback*, is a practice in which a referral source gets a fee for making a referral. Although common in business and law and some segments of medicine, it is more complex in mental health services. This is both a boundary and ethical concern because it indirectly draws a third party into the therapeutic relationship and can also create a conflict of interest (Koocher & Keith-Spiegel, 1998; Nagy, 2005). The 2002 APA Ethics Code (see also http://www.apa.org/ethics/) is very clear on the issue of referral fees; in Section 6.07: "Referrals and Fees" it states,

> When psychologists pay, receive payment from, or divide fees with another professional, other than in an employer–employee relationship, the payment to each is based on the services provided (clinical, consultative, administrative, or other) and is not based on the referral itself. (American Psychological Association, 2002, p. 1067)

A boundary concern is also introduced when a third party such as an insurance or managed care company; federal, state, or county agency (e.g., the Veterans Administration); or parent or spouse pays for the psychotherapy in part or in full. The concern is with the boundaries of confidentiality and whether the paying party can have access to clinical or other information. Similarly, boundary considerations are paramount in forensic, educational, and other settings in which a third party may be paying the therapist for testing and treatment. It is of utmost importance in all of the situations mentioned earlier that the boundaries be negotiated, if appropriate, but always explained and clearly drawn before treatment or assessment begins. Clients must be fully cognizant of who is paying for the services and who may have access to what kind of information regarding their assessment and treatment. Such informed consents must be clearly written, explained to the clients, and signed by them.

Initial fee agreement, billing procedures, and insurance reimbursement should be negotiated prior to or as early in therapy as possible. The following is a sample of the payment and insurance reimbursement paragraph that may be included in the office policies that clients receive prior to the beginning of treatment:

> *Payments and Insurance Reimbursement:* Clients are expected to pay the standard fee of $xx per xx minute session at the end of each session or at the end of the month unless other arrangements have been made. Telephone conversations, site visits, report writing and reading, consultation with other professionals, release of information, reading records, longer sessions, travel time, and so on will be charged at the same rate, unless indicated and agreed upon otherwise. Please notify Dr. XX if any problems arise during the course of therapy regarding your ability to make timely payments. Clients who carry insurance should remember that professional services are rendered and charged to the clients and not to the insurance companies. Unless agreed upon differently, Dr. XX will provide you with a copy of your receipt on a monthly basis, which you can then submit to your insurance company for reimbursement, if you so choose. Clients must be aware that submitting a mental health invoice for reimbursement carries a certain amount of risk and that not all issues, conditions, or problems that are dealt with in psychotherapy are reimbursed by insurance companies. It is your, the client's, responsibility to verify the specifics of your coverage. If your account is overdue (unpaid) and there is no written agreement on a payment plan, Dr. XX can use legal or other means (e.g., small claims court, collection agency, etc.) to obtain payment.

A new concern with regard to fees has been introduced in recent years with the advancement of technologies and the increased utilization of e-mail and Web-based communication and therapies. Therapists who use telehealth or telemedicine must be clear about how they charge and what they charge for. As mentioned before, telehealth challenges not only the physical reality of the place of therapy but also the parameters of time, especially with asynchronous communication. Because length of time to write or read e-mails is harder to determine accurately, many therapists charge a flat fee for a limited or unlimited number of e-mails (see chap. 8, this volume, for more details).

Bartering

Bartering, generally defined, is the exchange of goods and services. It has been part of humankind's culture since our beginnings, thousands of years before gold, silver, or other forms of money were introduced. Whereas most modern cultures, over time, shifted to the exclusive use of paper money and coin, and later to electronic and "plastic" currency, some agricultural and rural communities have continued to use bartering. Since the Internet explosion at the end of the 20th century, there has also been a significant reemergence of bartering practices via special online sites such as http://www.craigslist.org, http://www.barterco.com, and http://www.barterforless.com. Barter in psychotherapy and counseling is the acceptance of services, goods, or other nonmonetary payments from clients in return for psychological or counseling services.

Generally, bartering is more common in psychotherapy with low-income clients who seek or need therapy or counseling but do not have the money to pay for it. Bartering is also more common in certain ethnic cultures in which it is still an accepted means of compensation and economic exchange (Canter, Bennett, Jones, & Nagy, 1996; Koocher & Keith-Spiegel, 1998). Very naturally, bartering also becomes more widespread during times of economic depression, when either clients or therapists are in financial straits. Over the last few decades, some therapists have compensated for financial difficulties caused by managed care arrangements by incorporating bartering options in their payment policies (C. Peterson, 1996; Woody, 1998). Like fee-for-service and out-of-pocket payments, the use of bartering arrangements in place of insurance billing may increase client privacy and circumvent the inconvenience of preauthorization, audits, and delay and denial of claims (Hill, 1999).

Sometimes a bartering arrangement is in lieu of, or is part of, a low-fee or pro bono arrangement (e.g., chickens, fresh produce, or services provided by the client are part of the pro bono or low-fee arrangement). Canter et al. (1996) stated it well:

> Pro bono services, although certainly at times an option, may not always be possible, either because of therapeutic issues, the

discomfort or unwillingness of the client or patient to accept free service, or financial pressure on the part of the psychologist, particularly in economically depressed areas where many indigent clients may need psychological services. (pp. 51–52)

Many clients feel that if therapy is free, they owe the therapist some other form of compensation or they may be reluctant to confront the therapist or express negative feelings (Hill, 1999). Others may be too proud to accept services gratis. In these situations, to avoid embarrassment, bartering may be the appropriate and clinically preferred solution.

Most professional organizations' codes of ethics take a similar position with regard to bartering. On the one hand, they discourage their membership from engaging in bartering, but on the other hand, they permit it if it is neither exploitative nor clinically counterindicated and is an accepted practice in the community (for more details, see Appendix B). The APA Ethics Code has been evolving consistently over the past several decades in the direction of wider acceptance of bartering. Although the earlier ethics code (APA, 1953) clearly denounced bartering as unethical, the 1992 Ethics Code introduced a very cautionary statement: "Psychologists ordinarily refrain from accepting goods, services, or other non-monetary remuneration from patients or clients in return for psychological services . . . because such arrangements create inherent potential for conflicts, exploitation, and distortion of the professional relationship" (APA, 1992, p. 1602; see also http://www.apa.org/ethics/). It then defined the two conditions under which bartering might be acceptable: when it is not clinically contraindicated and when the relationship is not exploitative (Canter et al., 1996). The cautionary language of the 1992 APA Ethics Code has been deleted from the 2002 APA Ethics Code, which now simply defines but does not denounce bartering. A legal concern that is often raised with regard to bartering in psychotherapy is the matter of taxes. Goods and services received from a bartering arrangement are generally supposed to be reported as income for tax purposes. Breaking the law is not only a legal issue but also an ethical consideration, which in turn can become a therapeutic issue.

Possible Bartering Arrangements

There are several ways to structure bartering arrangements. The first way is using the fair market value of the exchanged goods and services. For example, if the therapist's fee is $120 per session, then a client's sculpture, with an independently assessed fair market value of $1,200, buys the client–sculptor 10 therapy sessions. Similarly, if a client has an established rate of $60 per hour for car repair, each therapy session will be bartered for 2 hours of car repair work. Rent agreements are also likely to lend themselves to a fair market value exchange whereby a client exchanges, for example, a $480 per month office rental to the therapist for four sessions per month. The second method is based on exchange of equal time rather than money. These bartering arrangements are based on an hour-per-hour arrangement, whereby an hour of a client's work is provided in exchange for one "therapy hour." The client's contribution to the exchange is measured by the time it takes him or her to carry out the service (i.e., car repair, writing a legal document, creating a Web site, cleaning the office) or the time it takes him or her to create, build, or complete an item (i.e., how long it took to knit the blanket or build the cabinet). The third, and more traditional, method of bartering is based on a simple agreement between the parties involved. An example of this type of bartering is the exchange of a chicken for a therapy session. In this arrangement, it is neither time nor money that ultimately determines the rate or type of the exchange but whatever is agreed on. The fourth way to structure barter is a combination of cash and barter, whereby the therapist and client agree on how much of the clinical fee will be paid in cash and how much by exchange of goods or services.

Bartering Goods and Services

As stated earlier, the most common types of bartering are for goods, services, or a combination. The following are closer examinations of some of these bartering practices. Bartering of goods is generally more acceptable and less clinically and ethically problematic than bartering of services (Koocher & Keith-Spiegel, 1998; Zur, 2004a). The reason for this is primarily that most often a fair market price or value can be established more easily and more objectively for goods than for services. As a result, clients are less vulnerable to therapists' influence and to risk of exploitation. Canter et al. (1996) added that bartering for goods may require less interaction than bartering for services, which may reduce clients' vulnerability to exploitation. However, even bartering of goods must be handled with care, as a particular object, such as a family heirloom, may have a strong sentimental value exceeding its monetary value. Bartering of goods also can become problematic if the therapist is not satisfied with the product received. Whether it is a commissioned pillow, painting, or maple syrup, there is always the possibility that the product may not meet the therapist's expectations or that the client may express his or her negative feelings by delivering a substandard product (Hill, 1999).

Bartering for services is a more complex form of bartering. Another variation of this form of bartering is arranging for the client to perform community service or a volunteer job for a mutually agreed-on local cause, charity, or nonprofit organization instead of the low-fee or pro bono agreement with the therapist. Thus, the client's contribution is being exchanged for therapy (Thomas, 2002). An example is when a very poor client, who shares the love of animals with the therapist, volunteers at the local animal shelter for 2 hours each week in exchange for weekly therapy sessions. Some bartering arrangements include a combination of goods and services, as in the case of a client who custom-builds a cabinet for the therapist's office. In this case, the client is an employee–designer for the therapist as well as the producer of goods (i.e., the cabinet). A therapist should use extra caution when bartering for varied dollar values, especially when a therapist's hourly rate is much higher than a client's. The reason for this is that clients may resent the discrepancy or view it as an unfair or unjust barter. Another combination is when a client owns an office building and rents an office space to the therapist, with the rent being bartered for therapy fees at fair market value of both.

Another type of bartering, which has rarely been mentioned, is guided by clinical rather than financial considerations. In this approach, bartering arrangements are geared to serve the emotional and economic needs of the clients and therapists regardless of their economic and financial situations (Rappoport, 1983;

Zur, 2004a). For example, a client who is a financially successful interior decorator wishes to replace a couple of poorly designed picture frames in the therapist's office. The therapist is aware that, in spite of professional success, the client still experiences low self-esteem and feelings of being taken for granted. The therapist agrees to the client's proposal to barter for new frames at fair market value, not because the client lacks money but because it provides an opportunity for the therapist to acknowledge the client and show appreciation in real-life actions rather than in words. Being taken seriously and professionally acknowledged by the therapist enhances the therapeutic alliance and significantly helps the client with self-esteem and professional pride.

Agreeing to Barter and Negotiating Boundaries

Regardless of the type of bartering arrangement, there are several ways that therapists and clients can meet, negotiate, and arrive at their bartering agreement. The simplest and most common is when the therapist negotiates the bartering agreement directly and in person with the client. This can take place before or during the first session or later on in therapy. Although not as common, some areas of the country have local trading associations that can facilitate bartering arrangements between therapists and clients who thus do not negotiate the bartering agreement directly with each other. These associations are composed of local merchants who agree to conduct business with each other through barter and without the exchange of money. The association standardizes the criteria and value of services and products, and its computer keeps track of the points or credits that each member accrues or dispenses (Canter et al., 1996).

Bartering in therapy is a boundary issue as it alters the usual, agreed parameters of the therapeutic relationship vis-à-vis remuneration and presents an alternative to the customary method of payment or insurance reimbursement (Gutheil & Gabbard, 1993, 1998; Thomas, 2002; Williams, 1997; Zur, 2004b). All bartering arrangements are at the very least boundary crossings. Although bartering of goods is more likely to constitute a boundary crossing but not usually a dual relationship, bartering of services also creates dual relationships. For example, when a client barters a sculpture in exchange for therapy, this does not generate another relationship besides the therapeutic one; it is merely a boundary crossing. The sculpture just replaces the cash, check, or credit card payment. Bartering of services creates a dual relationship in which barter introduces a secondary connection, most often a business relationship, into the therapeutic one. For example, a client who cleans the office or edits the therapist's book in exchange for therapy is involved in a business dual relationship because the client is simultaneously an employee and a client. Exploitative bartering is obviously a boundary violation.

Bartering presents a boundary challenge because it introduces a method, other than money, for payment and reimbursement for psychotherapy services and has been an especially controversial issue among ethicists and consumer protection agencies (Bennett et al., 1990; Herlihy & Corey, 2006; Simon & Williams, 1999; Thomas, 2002). Concerns range from therapists using their influential power to exploit clients to bartering arrangements that interfere with the therapists' objectivity and the therapeutic process (Strasburger et al., 1992; Woody, 1988). A major concern has been the complications that arise from determining the financial value of goods and services that are bartered for therapy. Traditional psychoanalysts view all forms of bartering as interfering with the neutrality necessary for transference and countertransference analysis (Epstein & Simon, 1990; Simon, 1991). Generally, the bartering of goods is clinically easier to negotiate and ethically more acceptable than the bartering of services because it often does not involve dual relationships (Canter et al., 1996; Koocher & Keith-Spiegel, 1998).

The questions around bartering for goods are primarily focused on the process of determining the value of whatever is exchanged as it is not always easy to assess fair market value. For example, even if a client's painting is exhibited in a gallery with a certain sticker price, it does not always mean that this is the fair market value of the painting. The gallery owner may have marked it up, expecting customers to bargain for a lower price. Or perhaps a client barters with an expensive item such as a sculpture, which was exchanged for 10 or more therapy sessions. Thereafter, the client or therapist decides to terminate therapy after five sessions. If the client were paying for sessions with cash, checks, or a barter item of lesser value, there would not be a problem, but a sculpture cannot simply be cut in half. It is important that a therapist and client discuss the potential complexities of bartering in general and bartering expensive items in particular. Articulating an agreement in writing can also be helpful.

Determining the value of bartered services is even more difficult. Whether it is housecleaning, editing, or designing a Web page, prices can vary widely. There are several additional issues around bartering for services and the inevitable dual relationships involved. The most common concern is when the client does not complete the job or the therapist is dissatisfied with the client's work (Woody, 1998; Zur, 2004a). Such dissatisfactions are likely to affect the therapist's attitude toward the client and therapy as a whole. To add to these complexities, there is also a possibility that clients may act out or express their negative feelings by producing substandard work (Hill, 1999). Bartering of services may also be more complex because a client may work for 10 hours for the therapist in exchange for 1 therapeutic hour, which, understandably, can cause the client to feel resentment or other negative feelings toward the therapist.

Additionally, a barter-for-service arrangement can turn awkward or difficult if it should become necessary to stop or disengage from it. When a client also acts as a house painter or marketing consultant for the therapist and therapy is terminated, the situation may become very complicated. One must be very careful when entering into any complex bartering arrangements that involve business dual relationships. Additionally, there is the scenario in which the client–employee is injured while providing the bartered service to the therapist–employer. It is important for a therapist who employs a client as part of a bartering arrangement to treat the situation as any other employment, and attend to such issues as a contract and insurance.

When entering into a bartering agreement, therapists must take into consideration the many details of the individual client, including culture, personality, history, presenting problem, economic hardships, profession, and other factors. As was noted earlier, artists and farmers are often more accustomed to bartering arrangements. However, bartering may be counterclinical with some clients, such as those with borderline personality disorder, those who are highly paranoid or suspicious, and those who see themselves primarily as victims. Similarly, the setting of therapy would determine the appropriate bartering arrangement. Whereas farming, ethnic minority (e.g., Indian reservations), poor, rural, and artists' communities are more conducive to bartering arrangements, most inpatient and urban settings are not. The nature of the therapeutic relationship is also an important factor. Successful bartering arrangements can enhance the therapeutic alliance and the probability of positive therapeutic outcome. However, a complicated or failed bartering arrangement can destroy therapeutic trust and nullify any chance of positive outcome from therapy. Finally, for a bartering arrangement to be successful, the therapist must be comfortable with the arrangement from a personal, cultural, and economic point of view.

Therapists must weight the risks–benefits of bartering arrangements very carefully and consider other options besides bartering such as low or no fees. They must avoid situations that are likely to lead to conflict of interest and any arrangement that is likely to negatively affect their clinical judgment, their feelings toward their clients, or therapeutic effectiveness. Therapists must make sure that risks are articulated, that clients are fully informed, and that the arrangement is consensual, fully understood, spelled out in writing, and part of the treatment records. Therapists must attend to and be aware of their own needs through supervision and consultations. Keeping meticulous written records throughout treatment is very important in the event that problems and complications arise with regard to the bartering agreement. It is just as important that therapists continually reevaluate the appropriateness of the bartering arrangement and change it, if necessary, through discussion with and, it is hoped, consent of the clients. If complications, negative feelings, or disagreements arise as a result of the bartering agreement, the therapist should discuss it with the client, seek consultations, and change it in a way that will be most helpful to the client and conducive to effective therapy.

Case Study: Cursed by Money

This is the case of a very wealthy client who openly admitted that she was "cursed by money." This client had never needed to work or pay her way through life and had all the time in the world to do as she pleased. On further exploration, she reflected that, in fact, she was cursed by money, time, and beauty. She spent her days shopping online and felt "stuck" in her large, expensive home. Money was always her way to buy love and effortlessly get what she wanted. Paradoxically, she was loveless, unhappy, and did not know what she wanted. After many months of mostly fruitless therapy, the therapist discussed the lack of progress with the client and her relationships to him and to money. It became clear that as long as she paid for the therapist's "love and care," therapy would not progress. As the therapist introduced the concern with lack of progress, he contemplated a possible bartering arrangement while considering the following: first, the client's wealthy background, empty life, and lack of major pathology; second, the big, East Coast city setting where bartering was quite unheard of; and, third, although there was familiarity and trust between him and his client, there was also a lack of emotional connection between them. Additionally, the therapist's existential–humanistic–developmental orientation was compatible with a potential, creative bartering arrangement. Lastly, he was aware that he was personally and culturally comfortable with a bartering arrangement. After lengthy discussions, the therapist and client decided that for 2 months, instead of paying the full fee for therapy as she had always done, she would contribute 1 hour of volunteer work at the local battered women's shelter in exchange for each therapy session. From a risk–benefit point of view, there was very little to risk but a lot to gain. This short-term bartering arrangement mobilized the client to be active in the world for the first time in many years and, as important, increased her trust in her therapist. As a result, she finally began to derive benefit from treatment (Zur, 2004a).

6

Space for Therapy

Interactions between clients and therapists outside the walls of the office, or what have been termed *boundary extensions* (M. Jones, Botski, & Gorman, 2003) or *out-of-office experiences* (Zur, 2001b), are the focus of this chapter. There is an extensive variety of such interactions: home visits to clients who are homebound or bedridden; home visits to families who do not have the means or are too disorganized to travel to family sessions at the office; and home visits that are part of case management, child welfare, or child abuse prevention programs, to name a few. Working with the homeless usually requires clinicians to attend to them where they are, on the street, in a park, or in a homeless shelter. Some clinical interventions are only possible outside the office space, for example, adventure or outdoor therapy; going with an agoraphobic client to an open space; accompanying a client to a dreaded medical appointment to which the client would not go on his or her own; consulting with an athlete–client at the gym, track, or field; or going on a brisk walk with a client who is depressed and medically noncompliant. A therapist may attend a client–artist's gallery exhibition or perhaps a client's graduation or wedding to support the client, demonstrate care, enhance the therapeutic alliance, or for other clinical reasons. There are many other clinical reasons to leave the office: Joining an architect–client to view his or her new building upon its completion, going to see the performance of a young client who overcame shyness and is appearing in a school play, and so forth. As mentioned previously, telehealth or e-therapy also takes place outside the traditional office walls (for more details, see chap. 8, this volume).

Our predecessors did not hesitate to leave the office on occasion. Freud analyzed Ferenczi while walking through the countryside during his vacation. Like Freud, Melanie Klein treated clients while on vacation and Winnicott took young people to his house to live with him while he treated them (Gutheil & Gabbard, 1993).

All out-of-office experiences are boundary crossings because they involve crossing one of the most fundamental boundaries of psychotherapy—that formed by the office walls. The out-of-office experiences discussed in this chapter are boundary crossings but are not dual relationships because they do not involve a secondary relationship beside the clinical one. Except for incidental encounters, all the out-of-office interventions discussed here are designed to enhance clinical effectiveness and client welfare; they are considered boundary crossings rather than boundary violations.

Home Visits

Therapists conduct assessments and treatments in clients' homes for clinical, pragmatic, and other reasons. Some clients cannot come to the therapy office because they are too ill, disabled, or too poor. Some families are too disorganized, do not have the means of getting to the office, or live too far away to bring all family members together for an office visit. Other families might derive special benefit from a home visit, whereby the therapist can observe the complexities and hardships of their lives and become familiar with the contexts of their family life, support system (or lack thereof), and neighborhood. In some cultures such as that of certain American Indian tribes, the home is a much more acceptable venue for mental health interventions than the medical office (S. J. Knapp & Slattery, 2004; Roberts, Wasik, Casto, & Ramey, 1991; Schacht, Tafoya, & Mirabla, 1989). Therapy or assessment at the client's home has been referred to as in-home therapy (Volker, 1999), home-based therapy (Boyd-Franklin & Bry,

2000; S. J. Knapp & Slattery, 2004), or simply home care (Slattery, 2005) or home visit (Morris, 2003).

Although some clients and families cannot make it to the office for a variety of reasons, home-based therapy offers some unique opportunities, such as meeting important members of the family and observing their community, including neighborhood issues (e.g., safety, crime, recreation, transportation, and communal support). There is an expanded opportunity to see what kind of people visit or drop by (Boyd-Franklin & Bry, 2000; Slattery, 2005; Snyder & McCollum, 1999) and the customs and rituals of hospitality. The therapist sees the clients' friends, who may not be likely to attend an office session. This might also lead to engaging the truly significant and powerful figures in the family. Getting a bird's-eye view of the family living situation, especially with regard to overcrowding, poverty, and disorganization, as well as positive aspects, can be invaluable for the therapist. It offers a chance to observe the family culture as it manifests itself in food, icons, music, and so on, and a chance to learn firsthand the family child-rearing practices. It provides a unique perspective on the family home almost as seen through the family members' own eyes. A home visit can also be a strategic clinical intervention and not one necessitated by the client's inability to come to the office or connect with the therapist via the Internet. Home visits reveal to the therapist an enormous amount of detailed physical and social information about the home not observable in office-based therapy (Cortes, 2004; Morris, 2003).

Most of the literature on home-based therapy has focused on interventions that are either part of family therapy (Berg, 1994) or some type of case management regarding abuse, neglect, or foster child issues (Morris, 2003, Slattery, 2005). Home-based therapy has been reported with American Indian families (Schacht et al., 1989), families whose problems did not improve with traditional outpatient treatment (Cherniss & Herzog, 1996), drug-abusing adolescents and their families (Erkolanhti & Ilonen, 2004), the chronically mentally ill (Heath, 2005; Menikoff, 1999), juvenile offenders in danger of out-of-home placement, and teenage mothers (Cherniss & Herzog, 1996), in conjunction with Head Start projects with disadvantaged families and families in extreme distress (Snyder & McCollum, 1999; Volker, 1999). Although home-based therapy is, in many situations, the only available option, there is no conclusive evidence of its efficacy in comparison with traditional, office-based therapy.

In the early years of psychotherapy when analytic thinking was prominent, home visits were not considered a valid clinical option for clinical–transferential reasons. However, with the cultural and civil rights revolution of the 1960s and the proliferation of psychotherapy modalities in the 1960s and 1970s, family therapists became more likely to conduct in-home therapy, and social workers viewed house visits as a routine part of case management practices. It took the passage of the federal Public Law 96-272, also known as the Adoption and Child Welfare Act of 1980, to make home-based family therapy significantly more common (Morris, 2003). The law was enacted partly in an attempt to avoid out-of-home placement of children and also to increase their safety through case management and home-based family therapy. As a result of the law, numerous programs were developed in which mental health and other professionals would work with families at home to help keep children safe in their own homes with their biological parents, siblings, and extended families (Bryce & Lloyd, 1981). The impact of the law went beyond foster child issues and, in fact, legitimized the shift toward increasing effectiveness of case management and child and family mental health intervention by working with the families within their natural milieu (Snyder & McCollum, 1999). However, the greater focus on risk management and defensive medicine in the 1990s has generally made therapists of all orientations more cautious and less willing to practice in-home therapy, resulting in frequent avoidance of in-home therapy.

The family doctor making a house call to an ailing child has been a revered part of American mythology and actual medical practice for a long time; however, this practice has not been emulated by most of the psychotherapeutic community. This is largely because of the early domination of the world of psychotherapy by the traditional analytic approach, which has been strictly office-based to preserve the neutrality and relative anonymity of analysts. One of the most obvious reasons for choosing home-based therapy is to treat a homebound, ailing, or dying client who is physically unable to leave the house (Gutheil & Gabbard, 1998;

S. J. Knapp & Slattery, 2004). This includes hospice clients, perhaps dying of cancer or AIDS, who choose to die at home. Then, too, there are such cases as the overwhelmed new mother experiencing postpartum depression or the acutely, and thus homebound, agoraphobic, paranoid, or obsessive–compulsive client (Morris, 2003; Zur, 2001b). Similarly, there are clients who are in acute crisis, which prevents them from coming to the office.

The geriatric population is growing exponentially, and the need for home visits is growing at a parallel pace. Untreated mental illness in older adult clients causes increased suffering and morbidity in the United States. Although more than 3 million U.S. adults age 65 and older need mental health care, half do not receive adequate psychiatric services (U.S. Department of Health and Human Services, 1999). Traditional, clinic-based mental health programs have not been sufficiently responsive to the needs of older clients who are mentally ill, a situation aggravated by physical, economic, and social barriers that may often prevent them from receiving essential psychiatric treatment. Access to such services by homebound, mentally ill, older adult clients is even more limited. In addition, these clients are generally more reluctant to seek out psychiatric care and are, indeed, less likely to recognize the signs and symptoms of mental illness. Frequently, concern with their physical disabilities may distract them from addressing their psychiatric needs (Bruce & McNamara, 1992; Kohn, Phil, Goldsmith, & Sedgwick, 2002). There is a deep need for innovative programs, such as in-home mental treatment, that reach out to older adults and bring treatment to them.

Family therapy has embraced in-home therapy more readily than most other orientations. Minuchin's (1974) work with families living in slums in the 1970s has often been cited as an example in which the home was the preferred therapy venue. His work also supported the inclusion of the larger community as part of family therapy, especially when the family is fragmented and a wider support network is available. Rueveni (1979), in *Networking Families in Crisis*, outlined the network process, which begins with a home visit to the nuclear family to assess the potential and feasibility of mobilizing the family's network of support.

Home-based therapy has been used extensively with ethnic minority clients and families, primarily because members of these communities often do not trust, and even fear, "foreign" or "mainstream" mental health professionals. There is often a reluctance to go to a strange place, such as a formal medical office, to talk to a stranger about personal problems (Schacht et al., 1989; Slattery, 2005). In addition, transportation concerns, distance, and accessibility prevent some low-income minority clients from getting to the therapist's office (Bryce & Lloyd, 1981; Roberts et al., 1991). Making a home visit to a client from an ethnic minority can be a key component in getting an important firsthand view of all the elements that make up his or her living environment and support systems. It is likely to help break the ice, decrease suspicion, and increase trust.

Outdoor or Adventure Therapy

The proliferation of drug rehabilitation, inpatient programs, and remotely located, alternative boarding high schools in the past couple of decades has resulted in a prodigious upsurge in the practice of outdoor or adventure therapy. This therapeutic approach is known by other names as well. It has been called wilderness therapy (Davis-Berman & Berman, 1994), camping therapy (Lowry, 1974), outdoor pursuits, and risk education (Ewert, 1987). What unifies these programs is that they are conducted in the outdoors, where clients are physically and emotionally challenged to overcome their fears and reassess their self-perceptions. They examine their beliefs in both their limitations and abilities and learn to rely on themselves and the group to carry out a variety of tasks assigned them.

Adventure therapy, as I refer to these various therapies, is mostly conducted in natural settings but can also be practiced in urban settings where there are indoor facilities for rock climbing or trapeze structures and rope courses. Outdoors, they most often include activities such as backpacking, hiking, biking, camping, canoeing, rope courses, navigating, vision quests (activities often conducted in solitude with physical challenges in nature and which may include fasting, spiritual questing, or both), rock climbing, and rappelling down cliffs. These forms of therapy are usually highly structured and are composed of individual and group challenges with a corresponding mix of individual risk taking, overcoming fears, and cooperating in groups (Schoel, Prouty, & Radcliffe, 1988). They have been used extensively with high-risk adolescents in boarding schools and drug rehabilitation programs; as an adjunct to therapy with long-term mental illness; in working with clients with mental retardation, substance abuse, phobia, withdrawal, or avoidance problems; rehabilitation of juvenile delinquents; families in crisis; and the hearing impaired (e.g., Banaka & Young, 1985; Gass, 1993; Glass & Shoffner, 2001; Herbert, 1996)

Participation in activities such as backpacking or rock climbing does not constitute adventure-based counseling by itself. Adventure therapy is differentiated from recreation or physical fitness in that it is geared specifically to eliciting therapeutic change and, like most clinical interventions, is designed for the purpose of changing one's affect, behavior, or cognition. There are six qualities that generally characterize adventure therapy: (a) establishing individual and group goals, (b) building trust among participants, (c) providing activities that challenge and elicit fear or stress, (d) participating in activities requiring problem-solving abilities, (e) participating in activities that are fun to do, and (f) having a peak experience that is the culmination of the program (Schoel et al., 1988). Adventure therapy is based on highly structured, carefully planned, sequential, challenging activities in which each activity has a specific goal that often must be articulated and achieved before the next activity takes place. Overcoming one's apprehensions, faulty cognitions, and perceptions of limitations by taking risks and relying on others is often the most essential part of these therapies. The outdoor setting is essential because such physical and emotional challenges are obviously impossible within the boundaries of the office.

Clinical Interventions Not Possible in the Office

There are many situations in which interventions are apt to be much more effective if they are conducted outside the boundaries of the office, and some other interventions can only be carried out outside the office. Some of the most frequently cited examples for such out-of-office interventions are in vivo desensiti-zation in the treatment of phobias (Gutheil & Gabbard, 1998; S. J. Knapp & Slattery, 2004; Lazarus, 1994; Zur, 2001b). In these cases, a therapist leaves the office to go to an open space with a client who is agoraphobic or perhaps flies with a client with fear of fly-ing as the final step in the behavioral therapy-based, systematic desensitization intervention. Along the same lines, Gutheil and Gabbard (1993) stated,

> It would not be a boundary violation for a behaviorist, under certain circumstances, to accompany a patient in care, to an elevator, to an airplane, or even to a public restroom (in treat-ment of paruresis, the fear of urinating in a public restroom) as part of the treatment plan of a particular phobia. (p. 192)

Similarly, the "anorexic lunch" and the "bulimic family din-ner" (when therapists join their clients for an actual meal as part of the clinical intervention) have been reported by family thera-pists to be very effective for clients with eating disorders (e.g., Fay, 2002; Minuchin, 1974). Sports psychologists often accompany their athlete–clients to the sports arena to instruct, support, or observe the clients' attitude and, most important, performance (M. B. Anderson, Van Raalte, & Brewer, 2001; Moore, 2003). When treating a client's complicated grief over a deceased spouse, par-ent, or child, it may be clinically indicated for the therapist to accompany the client to the funeral or cemetery, if the client re-quests it and it is clear that the client would not or could not go on his or her own.

Working with chronically mentally ill clients outside the office has also been reported quite frequently. This might include walk-ing on nature trails, going for a ride in a car, or just sitting on a bench in a nearby park. Clients who have been diagnosed with anxiety or bipolar disorders or schizophrenia are often too agi-tated to spend an entire session in the office. Walking and talking seem to be effective with some of these clients as they neither feel confined to the office nor feel a need to face the therapist but rather are able to walk side by side with the therapist and can be help-fully distracted by the passing scene (Banaka & Young, 1985; Heath, 2005; Zur, 2001a). Working with restless or defiant adolescents in the confines of the office has also been reported to be challenging. Robin Williams, playing the therapist in the movie *Good Will Hunting* (Van Sant, Damon, & Affleck, 1997), decided to effectively break the ice by taking the unusually resistant and distrustful young client, played by Matt Damon, to the riverbank for a walk.

Leaving the office, like any boundary crossing, requires special attention to how the client may perceive the intervention and how it may affect the therapeutic relationship. I had a very despondent, athletic, adolescent male client who had maintained a hostile silence for a couple of months during therapy. Finally, seeking a way to break through to him, I scheduled a meeting at the local gym to play basketball. Meeting on the basketball court and sharing the love of the game melted the client's reserve and helped him to open up and actively participate in therapy for the next few weeks. However, about a month later the client pushed the therapeutic boundary further and chose to join the recreation league in which I played regularly. His clear intent was to develop a close, social relationship. My subsequent attempt to contain the therapeutic relationship and avoid counterindicated dual relationships resulted in the client's feeling that he had been led on and betrayed. The unintentional and unexpected outcome resulted in the rupture of the therapeutic relationship and the abrupt and premature termination of therapy. One must take into consideration that boundary crossing always involves some level of risk that may arise from a client's view or interpretation of the boundary crossing as an invitation for a social or even sexual relationship (S. J. Knapp & VandeCreek, 2006).

There are additional clinical exchanges, not mentioned already, that cannot be conducted in the office. These include hospital visits, in which the sessions are conducted neither at the psychotherapy office nor at the client's home. Another example is working as a military psychologist on an aircraft carrier or at a military base (e.g., Johnson, Ralph, & Johnson, 2005). In these situations, the psychologist is likely to treat the client, as necessary, wherever he or she is. This can be on deck, in the mess hall or engine room, in the client's living quarters, or even on the battlefield. Aircraft carriers, in particular, do not have space to spare, and psychologists may not even have an office. Psychiatric crisis teams obviously are not restricted to the office or the client's home (Heath, 2005) but instead are trained to meet the clients wherever they may be, whether it is on the street or under a bridge.

Ceremonies, Rituals, and Life Transitions

Besides the situations in which clients cannot come to the office or the treatment plan seems to suggest an out-of-office intervention, there are other situations in which the therapist's decision to leave the office is therapeutically and clinically valid. The therapist may accept invitations to attend significant life transitions and rituals or celebrations in clients' lives. Attending the wedding of a couple who finally decided to get married after many tumultuous years of premarital therapy and attending the graduation of a client who never thought he would complete his studies are some examples. In their national survey, Borys and Pope (1989) reported that more than a third of the therapists stated that they accept invitations to special occasions with a few or more clients. M. Jones et al. (2003) reported that extending the boundaries beyond the office was rated as significantly beneficial by gay, lesbian, and bisexual clients. Celebrating and otherwise affirming clients' lives and accomplishments may be an important attestation for those clients who experience low self-esteem and have lacked external validation or the experience of celebrations throughout their lives. Additional examples include attending the first performance in a school play of an adolescent girl who, with the help of therapy, overcame her fear of public speaking; viewing the one-man show of a client–sculptor who finally conquered a severe artist's block; and going with a landscape architect, who had beaten drug addiction and depression, to view the prize-winning garden he designed and planted. Such special efforts on the part of the therapist have been reported to significantly increase therapeutic alliance and therapeutic effectiveness (Lazarus & Zur, 2002).

There are other events that warrant leaving the office. As mentioned earlier, therapists who work with clients from different cultures inevitably join some of the rituals, ceremonies, or celebrations because refusing to do so may cause irreparable damage to the therapeutic alliance, may nullify trust, and is likely to render therapy ineffective.

Giving or Getting a Ride

Giving a ride to a nearby bus or subway station to a client who does not have access to transportation or taking the client home on a rainy day is another rather common out-of-office experience (Fay, 2002; Lazarus, 1994). On the other side of the couch, over a third of the therapists surveyed by Pope, Tabachnick, and Keith-Spiegel (1987) reported to very occasionally asking their clients for favors such as a ride home. Such considerate acts fall under the aegis of common courtesy and probably do not require therapeutic examination despite the fact that a boundary is being crossed, unless, of course, such favors become problematic (e.g., demanded, expected, viewed as a sexual advance, etc.).

Incidental Encounters

Incidental encounters have also been referred to as chance encounters or chance extratherapeutic encounters and are defined as unplanned, random, or unexpected encounters between the therapist and a current client that take place outside the therapist's office. As discussed previously, incidental encounters are a common and unavoidable occurrence in rural areas, small towns, and university and college campuses (Barnett & Yutrzenka, 1994; Campbell & Gordon, 2003; Hargrove, 1986; Hyman, 2002; Nickel, 2004; Schank & Skovholt, 1997; Sharkin, 1995; Sterling, 1992; Stockman, 1990). Incidental or chance encounters are also not extraordinary in small enclaves within larger metropolitan areas such as political, gay male and lesbian, disabled, deaf, ethnic, or church communities (Guthmann & Sandberg, 2002; Kessler & Waehler, 2005; Llewellyn, 2002; Schacht et al., 1989; A. J. Smith, 1990). Such encounters are inevitable in the practice of sport psychology (Moore, 2003) and police psychology (Zelig, 1988), which operate in specific milieus, and in the military, especially on distant or isolated bases and aircraft carriers (Johnson, 1995; Johnson et al.,

2005; Zur & Gonzalez, 2002). Clinicians in these communities and settings randomly and frequently chance upon their clients in a wide variety of venues.

The earliest investigation into chance encounters was conducted by Glover (1940), a psychoanalyst, who called these encounters "extramural" contact. Like Glover, most other psychoanalytically oriented authors focus on the transference ramifications of such encounters (Sharkin & Birky, 1992) and, in general, view them as negatively affecting the clients and disruptive to the analytic process (Strean, 1981; Tarnower, 1966). Diverging from the analytic stance on the disruption of transference analysis caused by chance encounters, I assert that meeting outside the office does not necessarily nullify or negatively affect transference analysis, but instead the transferential reaction is more reality-based and provides more "grist" for the transference mill (Zur, 2000).

Chance encounters in college and university communities have received extensive attention. Given that most therapists in colleges and university mental health centers are also students or professors, that the counseling center and student housing are often located on campus, and the insular nature of university and college campuses, incidental encounters are common and unavoidable (Grayson, 1986; Harris, 2002; Hyman, 2002; Sharkin, 1995). Sports events, departmental social gatherings, graduations, and other campus ceremonies significantly increase the probability of chance encounters between therapists and clients in these settings.

Most of the concerns with chance encounters on campuses have focused on the issue of confidentiality. Contrary to a commonly held belief, Pulakos (1994) reported that students are not as concerned about confidentiality as their therapists are and, in fact, wanted more interaction, not less, when they accidentally encounter their therapists on campus. Sharkin (1995) pointed out that therapists avoiding interactions might inadvertently expose the therapeutic relationship rather than protect its confidentiality. In dealing with chance encounters, when possible, and in situations in which such encounters are expected, talking to clients and taking precautions are extremely important. These precautions usually involve discussing the possibility of accidental encounters with the clients at the beginning of therapy and understanding clients' preferred ways of handling them. Intake material and informed consent can also prepare clients for an inevitable, incidental encounter.

When encountering a client in public, it is important to take the cue from the client before choosing to ignore or address the client. Discussing incidental encounters with clients in subsequent therapy sessions can be beneficial; however, routine or brief encounters usually may not merit any lengthy discussion. The nature and importance of such discussions depends on the client's personality, presenting problem, and culture; the setting in which therapy takes place; the nature of the therapeutic relationship; the therapeutic orientation used; and the therapist's values and attitude toward such encounters.

Contexts of Therapy

To comprehend the meaning and propriety of clinical and other encounters outside the traditional office, one must examine four basic aspects of such encounters: clients, settings, therapy, and therapists. (Refer to chap. 3, this volume, for a more detailed discussion.)

Client factors including age, gender, culture, health, mobility, and living conditions are among the issues determining whether therapy may take place in the office or outside of it. For example, as was noted earlier, Native Americans may prefer to be visited at home and to have the therapists meet their elders prior to any clinical encounter. Clients who are homebound, unless they prefer phone or online therapy, must be attended to at their own homes. The client's safety is also of concern in out-of-office interventions. Situations may conceivably develop with clients who become acutely panicked, anxious, psychotic, or paranoid while on a walk or anywhere outside the office. Therapists who leave the safety of the office environment are inevitably exposing themselves and their clients to increased unpredictability and possibility of surprise. Of course, interventions outside the office may not be clinically advised for certain types of clients. These include clients who are acutely paranoid or psychotic, reckless, violent, volatile, or dangerous to themselves or others. Clients who express sexual attraction to their therapists, clients who tend to sexualize relationships, or clients who may require clearly articulated and enforced boundaries may benefit more from only-in-the-office forms of therapy.

There are numerous settings in which client–therapist interactions are inherently outside the traditional office. This includes home-based therapy, psychiatric emergency services, adventure therapy, and many forms of case management programs for child abuse, the mentally ill, and the homeless. Another issue when considering setting factors is safety. Visiting an unsafe neighborhood may pose a threat to therapists, especially if they are unfamiliar with the neighborhood and the local culture. Adventure therapy with its physical challenges and risks always includes built-in safety considerations (Gass, 1993). Whereas backups, cell phones, first-aid kits, and contingency plans are often available and established ahead of time in the office setting, more careful contingency plans must be constructed for encounters outside the office.

The various clinical strategies used when intervening outside the office, like most therapeutic interventions, are closely related to therapists' clinical orientations. As a result, there is very little agreement among psychotherapists from different orientations regarding the clinical significance and importance of such interventions. As discussed previously, social workers, adventure or nature therapists, case-management-based therapists, and family therapists endorse interventions outside the office. Analytically oriented therapists who emphasize keeping the analyst's anonymity and therapeutic boundaries clear, consistent, and distant obviously are not likely to initiate out-of-office contact. Similarly, the effect of incidental encounters on the therapeutic frame is a concern for almost all psychoanalysts and psychoanalytically oriented therapists (Epstein & Simon, 1990; Gody, 1996; Langs, 1982; Simon, 1991; Tarnower, 1966). Differing from the analytic tradition, humanistic psychology has its own very distinct view of boundary crossing, including leaving the office, incidental encounters, and dual relationships. Representing the humanistic view, Jourard (1971b) admitted that he does not hesitate to play a game of handball with a client or make a home visit if it enhances the therapeutic relationship. Behavioral and cognitive–behavioral therapists would also support leaving the office for clinical reasons such as going to the zoo to deal with a fear of snakes or driving with a fearful client over a bridge (Gutheil & Gabbard, 1993; Lazarus, 1998). Many feminist therapists support any therapist–client interactions that reduce the traditional doctor–patient power differential and increase familiarity (Feminist Therapy Institute, 1987; Greenspan, 1995; Herlihy & Corey, 2006; Zur, 2001b). Culture-sensitive therapists and those who work with adolescents, the chronically mentally ill, the disabled, and the disadvantaged emphasize flexibility and respect for clients' traditions, culture, and economic needs (e.g., Schacht et al., 1989). They endorse, when appropriate, home visits, going on hikes, and accepting clients' invitations to important rituals or ceremonies.

Therapists' factors also play a role in the decision to leave the office. Obviously, psychiatric emergency, case management, child abuse assessment, and outdoor therapy require specialized training. In-home therapy also requires some specialized training so the clinician will be prepared to deal with the unexpected and, at times, chaotic situations often involved in home visits. Therapists who work in settings in which incidental encounters are frequent must be trained to deal with them appropriately. Beyond training, a therapist's style, personality, and values are also relevant to his or her comfort level with leaving the office or encountering clients outside the office. Therapists who systematically incorporate communal and cultural values into therapy are more likely to engage in home visits and to attend cultural rituals and ceremonies. Similarly, it is more likely that outgoing therapists, or those who feel comfortable in the outdoors, will use a nature hike on a nearby trail with a restless adolescent or a depressed client. Additionally, the safety of the psychotherapist in the course of home-based therapy, psychiatric emergencies, or working with mentally ill homeless clients is an important consideration. Female therapists, for example, have reported fearing for their physical safety when visiting a home in which domestic violence has been reported (Volker, 1999).

Confidentiality and Other Considerations in Alternative Therapy Settings

Practicing outside the traditional office walls presents therapists with a number of challenges. These include challenges to confidentiality and privacy, start and end of sessions, and who may be part of therapy or is privy to the session.

The confidentiality concern is that encounters between therapists and clients during home-based therapy or incidental encounters can expose the therapeutic relationship to others in the community without the knowledge, consent, or control of either therapist or client. Some of the concern with confidentiality stems from a lack of differentiation between *privacy* and *confidentiality*. An anorexic lunch, adventure therapy, a home visit, or attending a wedding is obviously not as private an interaction as an office visit. However, lack of privacy does not mean violation of confidentiality, as these nonprivate, out-of-office encounters do not necessarily reveal any confidential clinical information. It is also important to remember that, ultimately, it is the clients' right to determine if they are comfortable with public knowledge of the therapeutic relationship; one of my clients, for example, openly acknowledged my therapeutic role during a wedding ceremony (Zur, 2001b).

Home-based therapy presents a number of challenges to the privacy of the communication between therapist and client. Neighbors, friends, and additional family members who may drop by the house or join a session or be invited by some family members to join the session are then privy to confidential communications. Although these additional people are present at the therapy session with the permission of the family, or at least some family members, this situation still stretches the concept of privacy and confidentiality beyond the traditional, professional view, and these concerns must be discussed ahead of time, when possible, or at the time of the session with all relevant family members.

Another challenge is determining or setting the length of sessions and the beginning and ending time of sessions or clinical encounters. These are often not under the control of the therapist during home visits, attending a wedding or funeral, walking on a trail, or participating in adventure therapy. Although sometimes the therapist can determine the beginning of the therapeutic encounter, this is not always true for the end of sessions. In family-based, home therapy, some family members may have to leave or choose to leave in the middle of a session, whereas others may respond to a phone call or a knock on the door, which may cause them to leave the session. Therapists who choose to join clients in rituals, ceremonies, and various public events have no control over how long these may last. Similarly, adventure therapy often takes unexpected turns that do not conform to the 50-minute or any other predetermined time frame.

There can also be uncertainty in determining who is and is not part of a certain clinical encounter once the therapist leaves the office and conducts therapy in a client's home or in a public place. Conducting therapy at the client's home requires that the therapist exhibit flexibility and tolerance for the unpredictable. Even when only the immediate family has been scheduled for a session, a curious or interested aunt or uncle may decide to participate, or a boyfriend may decide to "check out the home shrink." Experienced therapists expect such unexpected changes, and many view such capricious changes as part of the assessment and intervene according to what is presented and who is present. Although these unforeseen events can add richness to the session, they can also pose difficult challenges, as in the case when the intruding boyfriend or relative proves to be abusive, violent, or controlling.

While attending a school play, ritual, graduation, or medical appointment, the therapist has no control over who is part of the occasion. Whenever therapy is conducted in public, even with every hope of privacy, there is no way to predict when a friend or acquaintance may interrupt or even spontaneously take part.

Ethics, Standard of Care, Current Procedural Terminology, and Risk Management Considerations

Professional associations' codes of ethics such as that of the American Psychological Association (2002; http://www.apa.org/ethics/) Ethics Code, do not directly address the concerns of out-of-office interventions. Home-based therapy, outdoor intervention, and in vivo exposure, like any other out-of-office intervention that is part of a treatment plan, are clearly within the standard of care of behavioral, family, adventure, humanistic, group, and other nonanalytic therapies (Lazarus & Zur, 2002; Williams, 1997).

Many types of out-of-office experiences have been assigned Current Procedural Terminology (CPT) codes and have been recognized and reimbursed by the insurance companies. There are numerous CPT codes that address different types of out-of-office experiences. Mental health home visits are covered under codes such as psychiatric diagnostic or evaluative interview (90801, 90802), health and behavior assessment (96150, 96151), health and behavior intervention (96152–96155), individual psychotherapy (90804–90815), and family or group psychotherapy (90846, 90847). Similarly, there are numerous CPT codes for hospital visits (99221–99223), hospice (99377, 99378), interventions that are neither in the patient's home nor in the hospital (97535), and case management (6034).

Those writing on the subject of out-of-office experiences have raised legal (Bennett, Bryant, VandenBos, & Greenwood, 1990; Strasburger, Jorgenson, & Sutherland, 1992), ethical (Gottlieb, 1993; Pope & Vasquez, 2001; Reamer, 2001; Schank & Skovholt, 2006), and clinical (Borys & Pope, 1989; Simon, 1991) points relating to out-of-office interventions and the potential for abuse, exploitation, and breaches of confidentiality.

Case Study: Hospitality With Strings Attached

A woman therapist was assigned by her agency to treat a poor and highly disorganized immigrant family. In the course of 2 months, there was not even one session in which both parents and all five children attended a session together. It was not for lack of commitment to therapy that they did not all attend sessions. There was poor communication and lack of planning, but transportation problems, drug abuse, and abusive relationships also accounted for the sporadic attendance. Different family members had invited her several times to visit their home as a way to share their appreciation for her hard work on their behalf. They explained that in their culture, hospitality was one the most important values and an important way to express gratitude.

Upon consulting with a senior staff member, a number of issues surfaced. On the one hand, there were a number of reasons to support such a visit: A visit seemed to be a meaningful gesture within the cultural context of this family, and visiting the family home could give her a unique view of the family home and its décor, religious icons, the neighborhood, the neighbors, the sleeping arrangements, and so on. On the other hand, the staff member and the therapist were not sure how safe the neighborhood was, in general, and more specifically, how safe it was for an Anglo American woman to be there on her own. Other concerns were how to handle unexpected situations such as the presence of the daughter's abusive boyfriend; how to handle being served ethnic or exotic food; or, even more complex, alcohol, if it were offered.

It was a complicated decision-making process with valid arguments on both sides. From a clinical point of view, such a visit could result in valuable clinical information; there would finally be a session with all family members in attendance; and the visit could increase trust and enhance the therapeutic alliance, which, it was hoped, would result in further compliance with treatment. However, safety and unpredictability concerns must be taken into consideration. In view of the nature of the family, with its cultural heritage and chaotic structure, a family therapy modality supporting such home visits, and the fact that the therapist was an Anglo-American woman without any prior home visit experience, it was decided that the senior staff member, a man experienced in home visits, would accompany her. The family was told that having two therapists conduct a home visit was a routine procedure of the clinic and family members signed a release of information so that clinical information could be shared with the senior therapist.

7

The Home Office Practice

The home-based psychotherapy or home office practice presents practitioners, clients, and practitioners' family members with a number of clinical and familial complications and boundary challenges. These complexities are unique to the home office setting and are mostly not present in a traditional psychotherapy office. Such settings are often less formal than the traditional setting. For the therapist, it offers the convenience of working from home but also injects a significant amount of self-disclosure, raises safety considerations, and causes some crossover of the professional and private life. Moreover, therapists in private practice are often quite isolated from other professionals, and the home office setting, although more connected to family members, can only increase such isolation because there are no colleagues next door with whom to converse, consult, or socialize between sessions, during lunch, or over a drink at the end of the workday. As for the client, who is invited to the therapist's home premises, he or she is privy to a significant amount of information about the therapist's family, living situation, and lifestyle. For family members or others who live in or visit the therapist's home, the home office setting may quite possibly present situations in which they encounter the therapist's clients.

Unlike the other chapters in this book, this chapter does not conform to the usual prioritization of client, setting, therapy, and therapist factors simply because the primary thrust is the setting and the attendant self-disclosure—a major therapist factor. There are, of course, also important client and therapy issues relating to the home office, and they, too, will be given due attention.

Home practice goes back to the beginnings of our profession. Freud, Jung, Margaret Mahler, and Milton Erickson are among many of our predecessors who have practiced, at least sometimes, from their homes. As mentioned before, Winnicott took young clients into his home as part of their treatment (Gutheil & Gabbard, 1993). Despite the fact that interest in home sessions has not waned over the years and despite the long history of home-based practice, there is a conspicuous lack of research, theory, and practical guidelines on the subject. In contrast, industrial psychology has developed a general work–family theory to describe the complex interrelationships of work, home, and family (e.g., Clark, 2000; Kanter, 1977) that is relevant to psychotherapy practices located in the home.

Therapists seeing clients from their own homes is a boundary issue because it involves professional relationships outside the traditional place of business and the blurring of the personal and professional aspects of therapists' lives (Gutheil & Gabbard, 1993). The home office arrangement invites clients into the therapists' most personal domain, their homes. It exposes numerous aspects of the therapists' lives to their clients that would not be exposed in a traditional therapy office. It also can easily expose clients to therapists' family members, neighbors, pets, or whoever else resides in or near the house and vice versa, although this will vary from practice to practice.

Home offices come in different formats and arrangements. Some offices are located in detached units with separate driveways and entrances, distanced from the main residence. On the other end of the spectrum are the offices that are located in the therapists' living rooms or other designated rooms within the homes. In between these two arrangements, there are many variations with regard to which entrances or which bathrooms clients use and what part of the therapist's private home they get to see. The ages of the people who reside with the therapist will also vary significantly, and this could affect these arrangements. The presence of young children or teenagers, who are often less conscious of physical and time boundaries, may also be more apparent to clients, creating not only more therapist self-disclosure (see also chap. 9, this volume) but potentially more disruption or background noise. Similarly, the presence of pets may affect the ambiance and boundaries of the home office setting.

The predominant concerns with home-based therapy include the impact of home-based practice on the efficacy of the therapeutic process as it primarily relates to self-disclosure, privacy, and unexpected disruptions and the fact that clients are invited into the therapist's private space (Woody, 1999). Additional concerns include safety and privacy for therapists and their families and the impact of the practice on the therapist's personal life and that of the family. This chapter describes the boundaries and concerns related to the home office practice. These include self-disclosure; managing time, places, and people; safety, privacy, and confidentiality; client factors; screening and informed consent; ethical considerations; and, finally, contexts of therapy.

Therapist's Self-Disclosure

The decision to see therapy clients in one's home depends on several therapist factors, such as the degree of segmentation or integration the therapist desires in his or her work–family life, as well as the amount and type of personal information the therapist is comfortable disclosing to clients. When a client comes to a therapist's home office, he or she will immediately absorb considerable personal information about the therapist, his or her family, and the home environment. In the home office situation, therapists inevitably reveal where they live, the general value of their houses, the sociocultural aspects of their neighborhoods, how well tended their homes and gardens are, and how their living rooms are furnished and kept (Pepper, 2003; Woody, 1999). Depending on planned boundaries, or inadvertent occurrences, clients may become aware of how clean the bathrooms are, religious symbols, their therapist's domestic partnership status, how many children their therapist has and how the children behave, or how the therapist behaves in relation to family members or pets (Maeder, 1989). The plethora of information, conveyed primarily via nonverbal communication, enables clients to construct a relatively informed opinion of the therapist's economic success, artistic values, familial connections, and even spiritual and other values. The Woody Allen movie, *Deconstructing Harry* (Doumanian & Allen, 1997), although true to the producer's exaggerated style, illustrated how a home office can unveil to a client the intimate details of a therapist's marriage. In this particular movie, Woody Allen is married to a psychoanalyst working out of their home. When she discovers her husband had had an affair with one of her female clients (whom he had originally met in the living room/ waiting room), she cannot contain herself. She leaves her client in the middle of the session, bursts in on her husband in another room, and roundly curses him for his transgression. The client, of course, can hear the screaming and every word of the argument from the couch. The movie illustrates how private information about a therapist's marriage and emotional life can easily be revealed to clients in a home office environment, especially at times of crisis.

When practicing from a home office, a therapist has a responsibility that involves a series of conscious decisions about what information or messages are communicated through nonverbal self-disclosure. This includes, among other things, whether clients come into contact with and get to know family members, which parts of the home are available to clients, or how and whether to display art, family pictures, or other objects that may reveal aspects of the therapists' values or personal relationships. As discussed in chapter 9, self-disclosure can be valuable and may not be avoidable; however, in the home office setting, therapists are additionally responsible for maintaining an awareness of how such increased self-disclosure might affect individual clients and their unique treatment needs.

A variety of unexpected events can arise at the home office. There may be children's fights, loud music, and interruption of the session by family members or unwitting neighbors and friends. As mentioned, children, in particular, are likely to cross boundaries, drawn by curiosity or when seeking the company, support, and help of the therapist–parent. The concern is that for some clients, such exposure can be too disruptive (Pepper, 2003).

Another category of nonverbal self-disclosure addresses the communication issue of *metacommunication*, in which an intentional or unintentional interpersonal meaning is received along with the literal message itself (Perlmutter & Hatfield, 1980). For example, the literal message "I work from my home office" holds the simple literal meaning regarding an office in the building in which one lives, whereas the metacommunication may very well be "I am willing to allow you into part of the personal space of my self and the elements of my own life."

Managing Time, Places, and People

Running the home office and the relationships between work, personal life, and family involves careful management of three components: time, places, and people. These three aspects are crucial in determining the degree of segmentation or separation and integration or incorporation between work and family involved in the home office arrangements (Ahrentzen, 1990).

The hours when clients are received directly affect the degree to which the home-based practice may interfere with family life. If the therapists' spouses or partners work during the day and their children are of school age, seeing clients during school hours is likely to cause very little disruption to family life. However, seeing clients during afternoon, dinner, or evening hours can have significant effects on families with children but will have very little effect if the therapist lives alone or the spouse is working elsewhere during the afternoon or evening shifts. If the therapist is working afternoons and evenings at the home, besides the fact that the therapist may not be present at dinner time, there are other effects: Young children may need to keep quiet, teenage children may be asked to play their favorite music at a much lower volume, and so on. Along the same line, therapists who work in close proximity to family members may be distracted by worry about possible disruption, reducing their sense of presence with their clients. Maeder (1989) reported on the effect of home offices on the children of psychotherapists. He described the distress expressed by adult interviewees recalling the problems of avoiding their parents' clients coming and leaving the home office. Some recalled with anger the limitation on their movements during the last 10 minutes of each hour when clients arrived for or left 50-minute appointments. Work–family theory (Ahrentzen, 1990) predicts the obvious: The less the family is required to adapt their behavior to accommodate the boundaries of the clinical practice, the higher the probability of individual and family well-being. On the therapists' part, they are most likely to be aware when their family members are present and concerned about intrusion of their family life on the therapeutic process.

The location of the office is a prime factor with regard to the successful operation of the home office. Segregated offices, which are located on another part of the property and have separate driveways, parking, and entrances, may result in very little interaction and interference between the home and work activities. However, home offices located in the living room or in a designated room in the house itself are likely to have a much more significant impact. Offices located within the house itself allow the therapists to interact with their family members in between sessions. This can be a helpful way to stay connected and in touch or can be disruptive because of the rigid timing determined by the therapeutic hours rather than by the flow of family life. When offices are located inside the home, therapists must take into consideration everything that the clients may be privy to and assess its potential clinical effect. These include family photos, heirlooms, art, and furniture. Quality, style, orderliness, or cleanliness, even the cooking smells wafting through the house, may all have an impact on some clients. Such impact does not mean that therapists must alter their internal design to fit their clients; it only means that they should be aware and conscious of the potential influence on their clients and integrate it into the wider clinical picture and treatment planning. Clinical records may include statements such as, "Client responded to the background sounds of children playing and dog barking with deep sense of sorrow for her own emotionally impoverished childhood" or "In response to hearing muffled sounds of children playing in the backyard, client expressed sense of gratitude for what he saw as being included in the family household."

Time and space significantly affect the degree of separation between people in the home office setting and how many interactions there are between clients and family members. Additionally, some therapists inform or instruct their children or spouse of the level of interaction they feel is appropriate or that they feel comfortable with. This can range from complete separation, in which clients and family members neither see nor hear each other, to a free-flowing interaction before and after sessions. Of course, different clients have different needs and desires, and therapists are equally diverse in the level of familiarity and contact they wish their clients to have with their family members.

Managing time, places, and people can result in an office that is, in terms of work–family theory, high in integration, high in segmentation, or along the continuum between the two (Kanter, 1977). Although this theory has dealt primarily with the general issues of complex relationships between work and family, it also has a direct application to the home office practice. This theory states that work and family, rather than being separate spheres, are better conceived as interdependent domains or roles with permeable boundaries. At the core of the theory are two dynamics: segmentation, which draws the lines between the realms of work and family, and integration, which keeps the boundary in place by allowing professionals to cross back and forth over it (Clark, 2000; Kossek, 2003). The concepts of segmentation and integration are conceived as a continuum rather than as opposites. The work–family model suggests that the highest degree of satisfaction for those who work at home involves successfully balancing the two specific dynamics.

Achieving a balance between segmentation and integration can only be done by carefully managing time, places, and people and paying careful attention to the personal preferences of the clients, therapists, and therapists' family members (Kossek, 2003). A general personal preference for structure places one closer to the segmentation end of the continuum and would manifest itself in a home office that is located in a detached unit with family members either not present or far enough away not to be seen or heard. A general preference for fluidity and ease of transitions would place one toward the integration end of the continuum and would manifest itself in a home office that is located in or close by the main residence where clients have some interaction with the therapists' family members. Research indicates that a "good fit" between the practitioner's personality, preference, or style; family members' preference and style; and the degree of segregation or integration practiced is the best predictor of work and family satisfaction. Conversely, lack of careful attention to boundaries between personal and work life has been associated with work–family blurring and negative consequences, such as work–family conflict, stress, depression, burnout, anxiety, and dissatisfaction with both work and family life (Clark, 2000; Kanter, 1977).

Safety, Privacy, and Confidentiality

Safety considerations are of paramount importance in the home office setting, which normally does not provide the therapist or clients with the same level of protection as a standard medical or business office. When working with potentially violent clients in a standard office, there are often other therapists, staff, or receptionists in close proximity. In extreme cases, therapists may resort to the use of panic buttons, the door to the consulting room may stay open, or another therapist may be present during the interview. These options are not readily available or even advisable in the home-based setting (Herlihy & Corey, 2006; Nordmarken & Zur, 2005).

Safety issues go beyond the therapist's well-being as the home office setup may expose children, spouse, other family members, or other people who live in the house and even pets to potentially volatile or violent clients. The concern with a dangerous client in the home office is that if he or she was not screened out on the phone or identified in the course of some other pretherapy interview, that client now has knowledge of the location of the therapist's residence and with whom the therapist lives, who lives nearby, and even the layout of the house. Screening for individuals who are violent, dangerous, paranoid, intrusive, or psychopathic or any client who may pose a danger to therapists or their families is extremely important in the home office practice. Such clients are never acceptable for treatment in the home office.

The particular dynamics of time, space, and people in the home office setting directly affect privacy and confidentiality. Most medical or office buildings are designed to offer a relatively high level of privacy. Homes are not usually built with such concerns in mind. Most obviously, people who share the home with therapists are aware that the therapists serve psychotherapy clients

(Pepper, 2003; Woody, 1999). Neighbors are also often aware of the type of business that psychotherapists conduct and, therefore, reasonably assume that people who show up for appointments are psychotherapy clients.

As in the traditional office, the concern with privacy and whether others can overhear conversations in the consulting room is an important issue. Soundproofing the home office and using systems like sound machines in the waiting areas are as important in the home office as they are in the standard office. However, if therapy involves yelling or other loud sounds that can be easily heard by family members, it can be a serious privacy concern.

Client Factors

Suitability of clients to be treated in the unique setting of a home is a matter to be judged carefully. Although this often less formal setting can benefit some types of clients, it is not appropriate for other clients. Issues of parking, entrances, and waiting areas are usually clearly defined in a standard medical practice but are often much less defined in the home office arrangement. Clients need to be informed of boundaries and respect them. They must honor instructions with regard to where to park and which entrance, waiting area, or bathroom to use. Therapists with home offices risk having clients access private areas of the home, either by accident or on purpose. Therefore, clients who manage boundaries poorly are not likely to be good candidates for home office sessions. These include clients with borderline personality disorder, those who have interpersonal or physical boundary issues, and those mentioned earlier. For the same reasons, clients who are highly dependent or reactive or those who develop intense emotional, erotic, sexual, or hostile attachments may also not be suitable for a home-based office configuration.

Some clients have reported feeling, initially, as if they were intruding on the therapist's private space, fearing that they were being asked to cross a boundary from a professional into a personal relationship. They sometimes also wondered about the professionalism of the therapist. If these feelings are dominant for a particular client's personality or character, the home office may not be suitable. In contrast, average and highly functional clients and those who can benefit from the warm and casual ambiance that home offices often exude and the significant self-disclosure involved are likely to be good candidates for such a setting (Nordmarken & Zur, 2005). Suitability can neither always be accurately assessed ahead of time nor clearly predicted from the screening process. Therefore, therapists must continue to assess the appropriateness of this location for clients' treatments.

Screening and Informed Consent

Screening of clients for suitability, safety, and possible threat is vital in the home-based office. Although the issues of suitability and safety are always part of screening in psychotherapy, they take on heightened importance when the office is located in the therapist's home. To assure suitability and safety for clients, therapists, therapists' family members, and others, the screening process must be more rigorous and effective than the standard one.

There are several ways to increase the effectiveness of screening. The most common way to screen is by means of a phone interview. Some therapists combine such standard telephone interviews with a detailed questionnaire that is sent to the client and reviewed by the therapist prior to setting the first appointment. Such questionnaires often include detailed questions regarding prior psychotherapy, hospitalizations, suicidality, psychotic episodes, domestic violence, criminal activities, criminal convictions, addiction, and use of medications. When red flags go up because of suspect responses regarding volatility or past violent, psychopathic, or criminal behavior in the background questionnaire, therapists may consider obtaining an authorization to release information from prior therapists and obtain additional information about the potential client before they decide to interview the person in their home. Carefully reviewing the responses and the collateral information can help therapists make informed decisions regarding the suitability of the clients to the home office setting.

Another part of the screening process involves acquainting clients with how the home office is organized. The therapist should explain what clients will or may encounter in the office itself and with regard to where the office is located, the other inhabitants of the home, and, when relevant, the neighbors and the neighborhood. Some clients may be allergic to cats or birds or flowers, and therapists should incorporate this information into the screening process.

Some therapists who work out of their homes choose to take referral clients only and do not advertise through public channels such as online directories or the Yellow Pages. Other therapists choose to arrange initial intake sessions in a local clinic or in a traditional medical or office setting and then transfer appropriate clients to the home office setting. Yet others maintain two offices, one at their home and one in a traditional setting and—after conducting an initial interview in the standard office—make a decision as to which location is most appropriate for the client.

Most home offices provide rather different environments from traditional medical offices or office buildings. The detailed discussion of these differences must take place prior to the beginning of therapy at the home office. At the minimum, clients should be informed verbally during the screening interview of what they can expect in the home office with respect to the neighborhood, parking, neighbors, family members, pets, whether the office is located in the house or in an attached or detached unit, and so on. Clients should know in advance who they may have contact with. Some may need to know ahead of time if they are going to share a bathroom with the rest of the family. Concerns with privacy and confidentiality must be discussed in detail, as these are highly important issues in psychotherapy. It may be advisable to incorporate a paragraph specifically about the home office within the informed consent form that clients always should sign before treatment starts. This is a sample paragraph:

> Dr. XX's psychotherapy office is located in his private residence, which is located in the xxx neighborhood. Please park your car in front of the house or on the same side of the street where the house is located. Please use the main door to the house; just walk in (no need to knock or ring the bell) and proceed to the waiting room, which is also the residence living room. Depending on the time of the day, you may en-

counter one of Dr. XX's children, his wife, or his dog. Please, let Dr. XX know if you have an immediate concern with this arrangement or if a concern arises in the future.

Ethical Considerations

From an ethical point of view, there is no injunction in any of the major professional organizations' ethics codes against home-based practice. Such practice conforms to the standard of care. The well-being of the client and preclusion of harm are, as always, the first consideration for the therapist. Woody (1999) raised several risk management considerations such as privacy and confidentiality. Consulting in the therapist's home is neither unethical nor below the standard of care but requires augmented sensitivity to the ethical issues of confidentiality, privacy, safety, suitability, disclosures, and informed consent. From the point of view of billing and insurance, it is ethical to treat the home office as any other place of service or any other traditional, professional office.

Home Office and Context of Therapy

The context of the home office, like that of any other psychotherapeutic venue, must be assessed according to the four basic factors: client, setting, therapy, and therapist. Client factors that are relevant to the home office arrangement have been described earlier. The home office itself defines the setting of therapy. Although not limited to extraurban environments, home office arrangements are more common and accepted in rural, poor, isolated, sparsely populated, agricultural, small, and interdependent communities where medical or office buildings are less common.

Therapists from all theoretical orientations have used the home office. Additionally, the home office setting is likely to enhance therapeutic alliance with clients who appreciate the personal, more welcoming, and comfortable ambiance it provides. However, some clients may benefit clinically from or need a more structured and neutral office environment than the home office provides. Finally, therapists' personality, culture, lifestyle, and living and family situation would determine their choice of whether to work out of a home office.

Case Study: A Challenging Setting

The therapist in this case was a nursing mother of a newborn baby working from her own home. During a screening interview, the therapist found that the potential client's presenting problem was depression, triggered by a recently discovered infertility problem. The home office setting was uniquely suited to the therapist–mother and baby as she could nurse the baby during the breaks she scheduled between clients for this purpose; however, with this particular client the question had become whether the home office was an appropriate venue for therapy. The home office waiting room, in this setting, was also the residence living room, meaning that a crying baby could easily be heard and, at times, seen by a waiting client. The therapist realized that this setting, which normally accommodated her personal and professional needs very well, might in this case be an obstacle to therapy. In a subsequent phone interview, the therapist discussed the home office setting with the client, disclosed about the presence of a newborn, and shared her concern that the presence of the baby might exacerbate the client's depression and grief surrounding her infertility. She told the client that she would fully understand if the client would prefer a different therapist and offered to provide a referral. The client seemed moved by the therapist's disclosure and concern and, after further discussion, elected to start therapy, reasoning that this particular setting, although challenging, might actually help her come to terms with her situation. The therapist agreed to accept her as a client but made a clear commitment to continue to jointly evaluate the situation and to change the course of action if needed.

Telehealth and the
Technology for Delivering Care

The technological explosion toward the end of the 20th century, with its widespread use of cell phones, e-mails, and more recently, Instant Messaging (IM), chat rooms, video teleconferencing (VTC), text messaging, blogging, and photo-cell technology, has changed the way that billions of people communicate, make purchases, gather information, learn, meet, socialize, date, and form and sustain intimate relationships. Like global, national, and cultural boundaries, therapeutic boundaries are rapidly changing as a result. Medical information about diseases, diagnosis, treatment options, and medications, once available only to medical personnel, is available on the Web to anyone with a click of the mouse. Medical services, through the use of telemedicine (also called e-medicine or Web-based medicine), have been keeping up with the technological advancements. Telemedicine has proliferated primarily with patients who either cannot access traditional medical services or who have no medical services in their locale. This is particularly true in remote and rural areas and among the bedridden, homebound, and those who cannot access medical services for physical (e.g., disabilities, hospice, brain injury), mental (e.g., phobias, depression), or other reasons (e.g., lack of transportation). However, telemedicine has also proliferated among those who simply prefer this method of delivering or receiving medical services.

The use of the telephone as an adjunct to face-to-face psychotherapy has been common for several decades. In the past, the telephone was primarily used in emergencies, crisis interventions, follow-ups, rescheduling of appointments, and other basic, necessary communications in between office sessions. Phone-based suicide prevention programs have also been used successfully for many decades all over the world (Castelnuovo, Gaggioli, Mantovani, & Riva, 2003). Compared with the general field of medicine, psychotherapy has been slow to implement technology in providing mental health services to clients even though cyberpsychology resources are purported to be effective and present low-cost, convenient, and supportive services to the online population (Derrig-Palumbo & Zeine, 2005; Maheu, Pulier, Wilhelm, McMenamin, & Brown-Connolly, 2005; Maheu, Whitten, & Allen, 2001). Many knowledgeable people believe that e-technologies will provide the means to connect disadvantaged people with telehealth and telepsychological care (Stamm, 1998).

Thus, technological developments have not only affected the culture at large and general medicine but have also affected mental health services. In addition to the more common therapist–client telephone contacts, increasing numbers of clients have been routinely communicating with their psychotherapists via e-mails (Derrig-Palumbo & Zeine, 2005; Maheu et al., 2001; Recupero, 2005; VandenBos & Williams, 2000). Moreover, millions of people have been accessing psychoeducational Web sites daily to acquire information about diagnosis and treatment of depression, bipolar, anxiety, and many other common mental disorders (Zimbardo, 2004). Technological developments and increased usage of Web-based communication technologies combined with the ever-increasing popularity of the Internet, plus people's mobility and frequent relocations, have also given rise to a new form of Web-based psychotherapy (Maheu et al., 2005; Maheu & Gordon, 2000). These new ways of delivering mental health care have been called, among other names, e-therapy, online therapy, telehealth, or Web-based therapy. They include the use of Web-based technology such as e-mail, VTC, IM, chat rooms, and audioconferencing. Some of the communication is synchronous, such as phone, chat rooms, IM, teleconferencing, or audioconferencing, whereby communication takes place in real time.

Other communications are asynchronous, for example, traditional e-mails, whereby the communication is sequential and there is a time lapse between sending and receiving communications. *Telehealth* is a general term and has been referred to as the use of technology to provide clinical services. It includes phone, e-mail, and other Web-based technology in conjunction with, or independent of, face-to-face psychotherapy. *E-therapy* is a more specific term and primarily refers to the use of text-based technologies such as e-mail. *Online therapy* encompasses any Web-based technologies for the delivery of mental health services. Telehealth, e-therapy, and online therapy have reportedly been used increasingly in assessment and treatment of individuals, couples, or families or in group therapy (Castelnuovo et al., 2003; Grohol, 1999).

A remarkable boost to telehealth was provided by the Surgeon General's 1999 report on mental health, in which a concern was raised that two thirds of people who need mental health care never receive it because they are too embarrassed or shy to make in-person contact with a psychotherapist (U.S. Department of Health and Human Services, 1999). The report went on to suggest that online therapy is a possible solution because the nondirect visual environment offers these clients a sense of security and a way to express themselves with less sense of shame or intimidation.

Some federal laws were passed in the new millennium that have affected teletherapy significantly. The first one was the Telehealth Improvement and Modernization Act of 2000, also known as Senate Bill 2505. It was designed to further legitimize telemedicine services and reimbursement and provide increased access to health care for Medicare beneficiaries through telemedicine. The second was the Health Insurance Portability and Accountability Act (HIPAA), whose regulations, in part, arise from the realization that digital records and online transmission of records and information are proliferating at an immense speed. These regulations attempt to provide privacy, security, and minimum transmission standards to reduce unauthorized access and alteration of confidential health records (Zur, 2005b). These regulations directly apply to e-therapy, which is based on electronic transmission of confidential medical data. Similar to online record storage and transmission, one of the major challenges of e-therapy is reported unauthorized access to medical records. Such reports continue to make headlines in the popular press. Anticipating the growth of telehealth, several professional organizations and states' licensing boards have developed statements, recommendations, and guidelines for dealing with the emerging field of telehealth (e.g., American Psychological Association, 1997).

Telehealth and Therapeutic Boundaries

Telehealth and online therapy practices challenge boundaries both around and within the therapeutic relationship. Telehealth or online therapy transcends the physical boundaries of the office as phone or Internet-based therapies take place in the elusive setting we often refer to as cyberspace. Nevertheless, telehealth is subject to exactly the same federal and state regulations, codes of ethics, and professional guidelines that define the fiduciary relationship in face-to-face and office-based therapy (Recupero, 2005). It must fall within the same standard of care. Therapists who use it must still define who is the client, the beginning and end of the period of treatment, charges and billing, and, when possible, length of sessions and, if required, provide information regarding the nature of therapy. It also requires the therapist to provide the basic disclosures with regard to limits of confidentiality, to avoid abandonment, to develop and update the treatment plans, and to terminate appropriately. Telehealth transcends not only the physical boundaries of the office but also the boundaries of states, jurisdictions, and even countries.

Additional boundary considerations have surfaced in recent years as more psychotherapists are being asked to provide psychiatric advice to anonymous members of the public via e-mail or in chat-room conversations. Similar boundary issues have surfaced when therapists' Web sites have provided medical information by simply posting it or via interactive technologies (Recupero, 2005). As the standard of care for face-to-face psychotherapeutic care is applied to online exchanges, therapists will have to establish a professional relationship before rendering a diagnosis or proposing a course of treatment online.

Additional boundaries that are challenged by telehealth are the boundaries of confidentiality. Soundproof office walls and doors, a noise machine in the waiting room, and locked file cabinets have a different equivalence in the telehealth realm. Cell phones, cordless phones, and e-mails are generally vulnerable to access by unauthorized people. Traditional e-mail, IM, and chat rooms, like any other Web-based communication, are particularly susceptible to intrusion, which raises significant concerns regarding the issues of confidentiality and privacy. Internet Service Providers (ISPs), for example, have unlimited access to all e-mails that go through them. Break-ins into private and institutional computers and servers are alarmingly frequent. Virus attacks can send private and highly sensitive e-mails to all e-mail addresses in one's e-mail address book. Although firewalls, virus protection, encryption, separation of clinical from billing records, and other means and technologies try to combat such weaknesses and intrusions, the fact is that Web-based communications are likely to remain vulnerable to intrusion and confidentiality thus can be compromised with relative ease (Grohol, 1999; Maheu & Gordon, 2000; Maheu et al., 2001, 2005; Rosen & Weill, 1997).

Telehealth introduces new elements to the discussion of the second type of boundaries, those that exist between therapists and clients. Contact between sessions takes on a different meaning in many forms of online therapy, as an ongoing dialogue via e-mail is a hallmark of e-therapy or text-based telehealth. However, in videoconferencing, phone-based therapy, IM, or other synchronous-type interventions, contact between sessions is clinically, and boundary-wise, similar to what might be experienced in traditional face-to-face therapies.

Fees and charges also assume different dimensions in online therapy. Many online therapists charge via credit card and in advance. As the length of sessions is not always defined prior to the therapy session, the charge is often calculated on a dollar-per-minute basis. There are many ways that therapists charge for telehealth services. Some charge by number of e-mails, others by the time it took them to read, or read and write, the e-mails. Some charge monthly retainers for limited or unlimited e-mails (Derrig-Palumbo & Zeine, 2005).

Also, with regard to the boundaries between therapist and client, online therapy is not concerned with such issues as physical touch, office seating arrangements, or physical proximity (see also chaps. 10 and 12, this volume). Whereas text-based therapy, phone-based therapy, and audioconferencing are not concerned with clothing, videoconferencing is. As to the matter of bartering, online bartering, in general, has become a highly popular form of exchange that may be relevant to online therapy in years to come.

Ways That Telehealth Works

Technology-assisted therapeutic activities can be viewed along a continuum of least to most extensive level of mediation. This continuum may include the following:

- ☐ Posting self-help and education material on the Internet
- ☐ Therapist-recommended online psychoeducational or online support groups
- ☐ Phone and e-mail contacts as extensions of therapy
- ☐ Audio- and teleconference as part of, or substitute for, face-to-face therapy
- ☐ Technology-assisted alternatives to face-to-face therapy (e.g., e-mail therapy, IM, chat rooms, etc.)

The following are examples of clients who are more likely to use online therapy than face-to-face therapy:

- ☐ A young man in a small town in the Midwest who wants to explore his newly discovered homosexuality would not dare to consult face-to-face with any local psychotherapist but would sign up for online therapy.
- ☐ Clients who are very shy in person and do not feel comfortable articulating themselves verbally but are talented, fluid, and creative when writing.
- ☐ An acutely agoraphobic client who cannot find a local therapist to make a home visit.
- ☐ A family scattered around the world in different time zones that would like to have family therapy via phone, chat rooms, or teleconferencing.
- ☐ Clients who do not have access to therapists who can speak the clients' first language.
- ☐ A prominent public figure who wants to discuss his or her infidelity or sex addiction but would not approach any local therapist.

☐ A deaf client who cannot find a compatible signing thera-pist and does not want to use an interpreter.

☐ A reactive, defensive, or easily embarrassed or shamed client who looks for nonverbal cues in others and is likely to impulsively react to them inappropriately.

☐ A client who wants to work with a therapist who travels extensively and the only way to maintain continuity of care with such a therapist is via e-mail, phone, IM, or chat rooms.

In contrast to those who are well-suited for the clinical use of telehealth, other clients are not suitable for this medium. These clients include those who do not own computers, are not techni-cally capable, cannot afford the technology, or do not like the tech-nology and therefore will not be inclined to use it. Additionally, clients who experience acute or debilitating paranoia, schizophre-nia, bipolar disorders, severe depression, acute trauma, or inca-pacitating anxiety are not likely to benefit from telehealth unless they find the medium safe and helpful. Clients who have serious difficulty expressing themselves in writing are poor can-didates for e-therapy but may be able to benefit from video-conferencing or phone-based therapy (Maheu et al., 2005).

Clinical, Ethical, and Legal Considerations

When considering telehealth interventions, therapists must pay attention to several clinical, ethical, and legal considerations. Ethi-cal issues include concerns with confidentiality and informed consent. Often-mentioned legal issues are concerns with licen-sure and practicing across state lines. Clinical issues that have often been cited are obtaining proper identification of the client and establishing therapeutic alliance. As was mentioned earlier, basically telehealth must conform to the standard of care, like any other mental health intervention. Furthermore, it has been argued repeatedly that the use of technology, by itself, does not require changes in basic clinical principles and practices. Essentially, telehealth or e-therapy neither alters nor modifies psychothera-peutic theories, techniques, and methods (Castelnuovo et al., 2003; Maheu et al., 2001).

Ethics codes of different professional associations have attended to telehealth concerns differently. The American Psychological Association Ethics Code (2002; see also http://www.apa.org/ethics/) simply states that, basically, therapy that uses telephone or Internet must abide by the same ethical guidelines as in-person therapy does. The American Counseling Association's (2005; see also http://www.counseling.org/Resources/CodeOfEthics/TP/Home/CT2.aspx) Code of Ethics devotes a separate section (A. 12) to "Technology Application," in which it spells out guidelines for telehealth such as limitations, access, informed consent, use of the Web, and more. The National Board for Certified Counselors Code of Ethics refers counselors to a special Web page, "The Practice of Internet Counseling" (National Board for Certified Counselors, 2005b, see also http://www.nbcc.org/webethics2). In its code of ethics, the National Association of Social Workers briefly mentions the following, under a section titled "Informed Consent:" "Social workers who provide services via electronic media (such as computer, telephone, radio, and television) should inform recipients of the limitations and risks associated with such services" (National Association of Social Workers, 1999, section 1.03, para. E). These ethics codes share the basic concern with telehealth that is outlined in this chapter (i.e., confidentiality, identity, informed consent, crisis intervention, licensing, billing, etc.).

Practicing across state lines is one of the most complex issues regarding telehealth in general and Web-based technology in particular. This is because the lack of boundaries and the global nature of the Internet are not easily reconcilable with borders that define countries or states. Whereas some states mandate that therapists be licensed in the state where the client resides, others allow brief practice across state lines. Some states have not yet articulated clear guidelines on the issue.

In a large national survey of mental health professionals who provide telehealth services, Maheu and Gordon (2000) found that 75% of those surveyed were providing mental health treatment and services in jurisdictions where they were not licensed to practice. Of perhaps even greater concern, they found that only 60% of those surveyed even asked telehealth clients about their state of residence. Finally, 74% of those surveyed "were uncertain or incorrectly answered if their states currently had any telemedicine or telehealth laws" (p. 485). It is of vital importance that all telehealth practitioners learn the relevant laws regarding telehealth in any jurisdiction where they plan to offer services (to include where the services are received) and to not provide these services unless appropriately credentialed to do so (Koocher & Morray, 2000; Maheu et al., 2005).

Therapists who exclusively use telehealth must have a detailed informed consent form, often mandated by their state licensing boards. However, when therapists, as most therapists do, use e-mails, cell phones, and faxes as an adjunct to face-to-face therapy, they may use the following disclosure in their office policies and informed consent form:

> *E-Mails, Cell Phones, Computers, and Faxes:* It is very important to be aware that computers, e-mail, and cell phone communi-cation can be relatively easily accessed by unauthorized people and hence can compromise the privacy and confidentiality of such communication. E-mails, in particular, are vulnerable to such unauthorized access because servers have unlimited and direct access to all e-mails that go through them. Addition-ally, Dr. XX's e-mails are not encrypted. Dr. XX's computers are equipped and regularly updated with a firewall, virus protection, and a password. He also backs up all confidential information from his computers on CDs on a regular basis. The CDs are stored securely offsite. Please notify Dr. XX if you decide to avoid or limit in any way the use of any or all communication devices such as e-mail, cell phone, or faxes. Unless Dr. XX hears from you otherwise, he will continue to communicate with you via e-mail when necessary or appro-priate. Please do not use e-mail or faxes for emergencies. Al-though Dr. XX checks phone messages frequently during the day when he is in town, he does not always check his e-mails daily.

Similarly, e-mail signatures should have a clear statement with regard to privacy and other relevant matters. The following is a sample of such an e-mail signature:

> *Notice of Confidentiality:* This e-mail, and any attachments, are intended only for use by the addressee(s) and may contain

privileged or confidential information. Any distribution, reading, copying, or use of this communication and any attachments by anyone other than the addressee is strictly prohibited and may be unlawful. If you have received this e-mail in error, please immediately notify me by e-mail (by replying to this message) or telephone (123-456-XXXX), and permanently destroy or delete the original and any copies or printouts of this e-mail and any attachments.

It is important to be aware that e-mail communication can be relatively easily accessed by unauthorized people and hence can compromise the privacy and confidentiality of such communication. E-mails, in particular, are vulnerable to such unauthorized access due to the fact that servers have unlimited and direct access to all e-mails that go through them. A nonencrypted e-mail, such as this, is even more vulnerable to unauthorized access. Please notify Dr. XX if you decide to avoid or limit, in any way, the use of e-mail. Unless I hear from you otherwise, I will continue to communicate with you via e-mail when necessary or appropriate. Please do not use e-mail for emergencies. While I check my phone messages frequently during the day when I am in town, I do not always check my e-mails daily.

An issue that has often been raised in telehealth is the question of verifying the identity not only of clients but also of therapists, including ascertaining the authenticity of therapists' credentials. Because of the anonymous nature of Web-based communication and how easy it is to disguise oneself, there are concerns that minors may illegally receive treatment or that clients who conceal their true identity may not be able to be reached in an emergency. Although it is rarely mentioned, as a matter of fact, even in traditional therapy clients can disguise their identity as therapists almost never ask clients to show a photo ID and, therefore, their identity is never fully verified. The identity of the therapist is an equal source of disquiet. Although it is conceivable that a therapist might hang a fake, framed license or degree in his or her office, it is not very likely. However, online it is much easier for unscrupulous individuals to pretend to have credentials or to pose as someone who does have credentials. The concern with the correct identification of clients is not limited only to the name, gender, or age but also extends to address and state. A therapist may be given the wrong information about where a client lives, which may result in a therapist violating state law by practicing without a license (Maheu et al., 2005).

Another matter of major importance in telehealth is dealing with crisis interventions and the need for therapists to cross the boundary of privacy to protect the client from himself, herself, or others. The telehealth therapist may neither know for sure the identity and physical location of the client nor have information about local emergency services even when the client's location is known. There is an apprehension that therapists may be aware of clients in jeopardy but cannot intervene because the location of the endangered or dying clients may be unknown. One of the most cited responses to the concern regarding crisis intervention by e-therapists is the long known efficacy of crisis hotlines and suicide prevention phone services. Established online clinics, which host a large number of e-therapists, provide the therapists with wide access to emergency services anywhere in the United States that can be matched with clients' addresses (Derrig-Palumbo & Zeine, 2005).

Last but not least is the frequently mentioned nature and quality of the therapeutic alliance, articulated in this book as one part of the boundaries between therapists and clients. In contrast to the commonly held belief among therapists, the therapeutic alliance established online is reported to be positive in a growing number of publications (i.e., Castelnuovo et al., 2003; Rees & Stone, 2005). The belief that e-therapy does not lend itself to strong therapeutic alliance would seem to call into question the intensity of emotional bonds shared by people who sustain relationships via cell phones, standard e-mail, IM, or chat rooms. Electronic communication allows both the client and the professional to fully reflect on issues discussed in previous correspondence. Unlike other helping methods such as traditional psychotherapy, e-therapy's strength is in the ability to explore and flesh out a person's concerns without awkwardness or the need to "think on one's feet." The lack of visual cues, such as body language, has been cited as a major barrier to the therapeutic alliance (Rees & Stone, 2005). However, the efficacy of blind therapists and the fact that traditional psychoanalytic therapy has placed clients on the couch specifically to prevent them from picking up visual cues from the therapists should provide some assurance that the lack of direct visual cues is not necessarily an obstacle to therapeutic relationships. Proponents of e-therapy have emphasized the fact that text-based therapy has the potential to significantly reduce emotional or instinctive responses and do away with reactivity to therapists' perceived body language. It has been argued that such intervention can increase the effectiveness of communication, as past communication can be accessed and referred to at any time, while eliminating unconscious reactivity and impulsiveness (Derrig-Palumbo & Zeine, 2005).

Guidelines for Using Technology in Psychotherapy

The following are some suggestions for ways that therapists can attend to boundary concerns raised in this chapter:

- [ ] Identify the client and obtain basic information such as full name, address, age, gender, phone, fax, emergency contacts, and so on.
- [ ] Provide clients with a clear informed consent form detailing the limitations of telehealth, in general, and confidentiality and privacy, in particular.
- [ ] Inform the clients of potential limitations of telehealth when it comes to crisis interventions and dealing with dangerous situations.
- [ ] Practice within your limits of clinical and technological competence.
- [ ] Have a crisis intervention plan in place, including ways to reach local emergency services and make referrals to local psychotherapists, psychiatrists, and psychiatric hospitals in the client's vicinity.
- [ ] Provide thorough screening when considering which clients may not be suited to this kind of medium.
- [ ] Have a clear agreement with regard to what is being charged, how it is being charged, and the rates and method of payment.
- [ ] Do not render medical or psychiatric advice by giving a diagnosis or proposing a course of treatment except to

those with whom you have established professional psychotherapeutic relationships.

☐ Follow your state laws, your licensing board rules, and
your state and national professional association guidelines
and practice within the standard of care.

☐ Screen clients for technical and clinical suitability for
telehealth.

☐ Telehealth is one of the fastest growing fields in medicine.
Update yourself on the latest research on telehealth.

Case Study: The Medium Is Not the Message

The male client, an engineer in a large firm, found a therapist in
his state via the Internet. He contacted the therapist by e-mail
and presented his problem as shyness and an addiction to online
pornography. The client clearly stated that he was not willing to
see a local therapist in person, as he was concerned he would be
recognized and shamed. Because the client seemed generally functional, emotionally stable, computer literate, and clear about the
modality of therapy he was seeking, the therapist made the determination that the client and his presenting problems were
suitable for e-therapy. The ensuing e-mail correspondence involved clarification of what medium the client preferred and
what technologies were available to the therapist. It also included
a few forms such as the general informed consent form, HIPAA
notice of privacy practices, and fee agreement and credit card
authorization that the client downloaded from the therapist's
Web site. Additionally, a biographical questionnaire, including
name, address, phone, and extensive medical, social, and family
history, was downloaded and filled out by the client. After a
brief phone conversation with the client that verified some of
the biographical details, therapy started. It included a series of
e-mails that went back and forth twice a week and included referrals to psychoeducational Web sites on addiction and shyness. The client submitted a weekly log noting use of pornography and other issues. The therapist used psychoeducational and
cognitive–behavioral techniques. Also, the client was referred
to well-established online support groups for those who experi-

ence shyness and for those who are challenged by addiction to online pornography.

As agreed, the client paid by credit card, monthly in advance, but used the therapy inconsistently. After communicating for a couple of weeks regularly, he would disappear for a week or two. He did not mind paying even though he was not using the services regularly. The nature and content of e-mails and the intermittent dropping out of sight indicated to the therapist that the therapeutic alliance was not very strong. In contrast, the addiction logs showed clear improvement with regard to his decreasing use of online pornography. Further inquiry revealed that the client's reliance on the online support groups for shyness was highly effective. He started going out more, dealing with his shyness more successfully, and even went on some "practice dates" a few times. Four months after the beginning of therapy, he stopped all communication, and the credit card payments stopped as well. The therapist's e-mails with regard to stopping therapy were not returned except for a short note saying, "Your services are no longer needed." The therapist followed up with a short e-mail acknowledging the termination of services, offering to provide referral if the client was interested, and stating that he was open to consider resuming therapy if the client so wished in future. Reflecting on the case in his peer supervision group, the therapist realized that the medium is not the message. The e-therapy with the client was not inherently different from therapy with other clients: Some do gain something from therapy, some are not intimately connect with the therapist, and some terminate unexpectedly. Even though the termination was abrupt and impersonal, with the help of the support group the therapist realized that his own need for a different, more comprehensive, and personal closure was not clinically necessary. He also realized that from an ethical and legal point of view, he must respect the client's wish to terminate the fiduciary relationship in any way he saw fit, as long as the client did not pose a danger to himself or others and there were no other clinical concerns regarding termination.

III

Boundaries Within the Therapeutic Encounter

9

Self-Disclosure

Therapists' self-disclosure refers to therapists' revelations of personal rather than professional information about themselves to their clients. Such self-disclosure has been classified as deliberate, unavoidable, or accidental. Deliberate self-disclosure usually refers to therapists' intentional, verbal disclosure of personal information, but it also applies to other deliberate actions such as an empathic gesture or placing a certain family photo in the office. Unavoidable self-disclosure might include a therapist's tone of voice, foreign accent, and a great range of other cues, as detailed subsequently. Home office arrangements inevitably involve extensive, unavoidable self-disclosure (see chap. 7, this volume, for more details). Accidental self-disclosure occurs when there are incidental encounters outside the office, spontaneous verbal or nonverbal reactions, or other unplanned occurrences that happen to reveal therapists' personal information to their clients (Knox, Hess, Petersen, & Hill, 1997; Stricker & Fisher, 1990). Narrative therapists have used the term *therapists' transparency* in a way that is similar to the use of the term *self-disclosure* in the professional literature (White & Epston, 1990).

Intentional, verbal self-disclosures include therapists' disclosure of information about themselves and also their personal reactions to clients and to occurrences that take place during sessions. These two types of self-disclosures have been described, respectively, as self-revealing and self-involving (Knox et al.,

1997). Intentional self-disclosure can be initiated by clients when they question their therapists about personal matters or by therapists who volunteer personal information. Clients' professional inquiries regarding the therapist's degree, license, scope of practice, experience, or fee are considered standard inquiries and are not thought of as self-disclosure. Clients' inquiries regarding therapists' personal lives via the Internet, stalking, or other surreptitious means can result in a client being privy to extensive personal information about their therapists, who may not even be aware of the amount of information available to their clients.

National surveys have consistently shown that most therapists are involved in some form of intentional self-disclosure. In one of the largest of such surveys, Pope, Tabachnick, and Keith-Spiegel (1987) reported that at least 90% of the therapist–respondents indicated that they engaged in self-disclosure behavior, at least on rare occasions. The same survey also concluded that not only do most therapists use self-disclosure, but more specifically, most therapists (89.7%) tell clients when they are angry with them and more than half cry (56.5%) in the presence of a client and tell clients when they are disappointed in them (51.9%). Pope et al. (1987) concluded, "Thus, it appears that the more extreme versions of the therapist as 'blank screen' are exceedingly rare among psychologists" (p. 998). A survey (by the same researchers) reporting on therapists who are themselves in therapy yielded similar results, with a majority reporting that on at least one occasion their therapists had told them that they cared about them. Over one third of the therapist–clients noted that their therapists had expressed anger toward them at least once, and slightly less than a third reported that their therapists had expressed disappointment in them. Similarly, about half of the therapists reported that they disclosed details of current personal stresses to a client (Borys & Pope, 1989; DeJulio & Berkman, 2003). Research on therapists who treated self-defined lesbian and gay male clients revealed that 63% of them were prescreened for gay-affirmative attitudes (Liddle, 1997).

Analysis of interviews with clients about therapist self-disclosure reveals that helpful disclosures occurred more often when clients discussed important issues (Knox et al., 1997). Disclosures were perceived as intended by therapists to normalize or reassure the clients and tended to be a spontaneous disclosure of personal information. The researchers concluded that therapist self-disclo-sures improved therapeutic relationships significantly. Accord-ing to research, clients who expected their therapists to self-dis-close have disclosed more themselves compared with clients who did not expect disclosure or whose therapists did not self-dis-close (Stricker & Fisher, 1990). Rosie's (1974) finding that more experienced therapists are more likely to self-disclose is consis-tent with Williams's (1997) observation that older therapists are more comfortable with boundary crossing in psychotherapy.

Self-Disclosure as an Ethical and Boundary Issue

Self-disclosure is considered a boundary issue as it crosses the interpersonal boundary between therapists and clients in the di-rection of the client rather than in the professionally expected di-rection of the therapist. Appropriate and clinically driven self-disclosures that are carried out for the clinical benefit of the clients are considered boundary crossings (Gutheil & Gabbard, 1993; Lazarus & Zur, 2002; Williams, 1997). Similarly, unavoidable self-disclosures that take place as a normal part of living in a small community are also boundary crossings. Inappropriate self-disclosure, which is done primarily for the benefit of the thera-pist, is clinically counterindicated, burdens the client with un-necessary or clinically irrelevant information about the therapist, or creates a role reversal whereby a client, inappropriately, takes care of the therapist, is considered a boundary violation (Gutheil & Gabbard, 1998; Zur, 2004b).

There are a number of concerns that are associated with self-disclosure. The most important of these is that self-disclosure is not done for clinical–therapeutic purposes or for the client's ben-efit but rather for the therapist's. Thus, the intent of the therapist is extremely important because it should be focused firmly on the client's welfare and should not be fueled by the gratification of the therapist's needs or desires (Barnett, 1998; Bridges, 2001; Herlihy & Corey, 2006; Mallow, 1998; Reamer, 2001). Several writ-ers have raised the concern that the therapist's self-disclosure should not burden the client, be excessive, or create a situation in which the client needs to care for the therapist. Most scholars and ethicists agree that therapists should not share their sexual fantasies with their clients (Fisher, 2004; Gabbard, 1989; Pope et al., 1987; Stricker & Fisher, 1990).

Risk management experts have raised the issue that ethics committees, licensing boards, or juries may look suspiciously on the fact that clients have considerable personal information about their therapists (Gutheil & Gabbard, 1993; Williams, 1997). These experts have observed that therapist self-disclosure has often taken place in therapist–client relationships that ended up in sexual or other unethical or illegal interactions (Pope, Sonne, & Holroyd, 1993; Strasburger, Jorgenson, & Sutherland, 1992). However, self-disclosure, by itself, does not necessarily lead to sexual transgression with clients (Stricker & Fisher, 1990). As with any other intervention, and consistent with the standard of care, therapists must document their intervention, including extensive clinical use of self-disclosure as part of their treatment plans. In the event that significant self-disclosure is used, the treatment plan should clarify how it is implemented for clinical reasons appropriate and specific to the client with that specific mental condition. When relevant, therapists' theoretical orientation should also be articulated, as many orientations support self-disclosure as an effective clinical tool.

Like any decision regarding boundary crossing, let us note yet again that the decision to self-disclose is based first and foremost on the welfare of the client. Intentional and deliberate self-disclosure is made under the general moral and ethical principles of beneficence and nonmaleficence—therapists intervene in ways that are intended to benefit their clients and avoid harm to them (American Psychological Association [APA], 2002). Applying these principles to self-disclosure means that intentional self-disclosure should be client focused and clinically driven and not intended to gratify the therapists' needs. When self-disclosure is unavoidable, as often is the case in small communities, therapists must evaluate whether such exposure is likely to benefit, interfere with, or affect the therapeutic process in any way. Self-disclosure, or what has been called self-involving (Knox et al., 1997), has also been discussed in the context of therapists' struggle to maintain neutrality and respond appropriately in cases in which clients were accused or admitted to being involved in child pornography (Lally & Freeman, 2005), rape, or other violent actions. In these situations, a therapist's spontaneous or involuntary negative reaction, although understandable, is likely to affect the therapeutic process.

Therapist's Choices in Self-Disclosure

A therapist's gender, ethnicity, age, physical characteristics, and foreign accent are self-disclosures that are unavoidable. Pregnancy is another example of a significant self-disclosure that is not by the therapist's choice (Schwartz, 1975), as are stuttering, visible tattoos, and obesity. Many forms of disability such as paralysis, blindness, deafness, or an apparent limp, missing limb, or visible scars also represent unavoidable self-disclosures. Therapists reveal themselves also by their manner of dress, hairstyle, makeup, jewelry, perfume or aftershave, facial hair, wedding or engagement rings, or the wearing of a cross, star, or other religious symbol (Barnett, 1998; Tillman, 1998).

Body language and numerous other nonverbal cues are other sources of self-disclosure, all of which are highly significant for the therapeutic exchange but are nevertheless not under the therapist's full control. In general, the client is often more attuned to nonverbal cues such as body language and touch than to verbal communication (M. L. Knapp & Hall, 1997). A raised eyebrow, recoil, nod, flinch, leaning forward, and hundreds of other subtle body language expressions give clients information about the therapist, providing fertile ground to project the meaning of these cues. Even for traditional psychoanalysts who strive to minimize self-disclosure, every intervention nonetheless hides some things about the analysts and reveals others. Aron (1991), writing for *Psychoanalytic Dialogues,* stated, "Self-revelation is not an option; it is an inevitability" (p. 40). The question then becomes not whether to disclose, but how to take into consideration the unavoidable condition of constant disclosure.

Another type of self-disclosure occurs when therapists are required or expected to share professionally relevant personal information. This kind of information includes telling clients when the therapists will not be scheduling appointments. The therapist may be attending a professional conference, going on vacation, having surgery, attending to a sick relative, or any reason that means being unavailable to clients for a period of time. Therapists vary in the degree that they may self-disclose the reason for the absence. Similarly, when therapists contemplate closing their practices as a result of illness, retirement, or relocation, they must tell their clients ahead of time and explain the general reasons. Treatments that take place outside the office often require therapists to disclose personal information. During a home visit or during adventure therapy, therapists may need to reveal if they are vegetarians or perhaps eat only kosher food. Similarly, during adventure therapy, cultural, religious, or spiritual orientations may be revealed through rituals and other self-disclosing behaviors. (For additional information on complexities of out-of-office experiences, refer to chap. 6, this volume. For more details on verbal and nonverbal communication, see chap. 12, this volume.)

The Evolution of Societal and Therapeutic Attitudes Toward Self-Disclosure

Discussions of psychotherapists' self-disclosures date back to the earliest years of psychotherapy. As early as 1912, Freud emphasized that "The physician should be impenetrable to the patient, and like a mirror, reflect nothing but what is shown to him" (C. Peterson, 2002, p. 21). Along the same lines, Freud expressed his discontent with his student Ferenczi's extensive self-disclosure with his clients (D. Smith & Fitzpatrick, 1995). However, Freud himself revealed many aspects of his personal life to his patients, shared his dreams and recollections of his early childhood with them, and gave them self-revealing gifts (Blanton, 1971; Goldstein, 1997). Departing from Freud's theoretical stance of self-disclosure, several analysts, such as Micael Balint, Paula Heimann, and Wilhelm Reich, have discussed the value of self-disclosure of countertransference reactions to the therapeutic process (Barnett, 1998). Adhering to Freud's view, the analytic and behavioral therapists who dominated the field of psychotherapy through the first part of the 20th century were in agreement that self-disclosure is to be avoided when possible.

The rise of the humanist movement in the 1960s advanced the argument that self-disclosure could be therapeutic and valuable (Jourard, 1971b). The feminist movement of the 1970s and 1980s added a political dimension, in which feminist therapists' self-disclosure was valued for its role in modeling and fostering a more egalitarian relationship between therapist and client (Brown, 1994; Greenspan, 1995; Simi & Mahalik, 1997).

The 12-step programs, used in many support groups and which are based on mutual self-disclosure have proliferated since the 1980s and 1990s. Such support groups have spread widely beyond alcohol and drug addiction to include support groups for survival of childhood abuse, disabilities, illnesses, victims of racism, sexism, homophobia, and a broad range of codependency groups.

The 1990s have witnessed a cultural shift whereby the public has become accustomed to intimate and detailed confessions on national TV by celebrities and politicians such as Oprah Winfrey, Kitty Dukakis, Elizabeth Taylor, and Patty and Michael Reagan. At the same time, *Oprah, Dr. Phil, Geraldo,* and *Donahue*-type shows have promoted extreme and often bizarre self-disclosure by people on TV in front of millions of strangers. More recently, so-called reality shows that promote uncensored voyeurism and uninhibited self-disclosure have burgeoned. These societal traits are best symbolized by the extensive and graphic transcripts of Monica Lewinsky's testimony on her sexual affair with President Clinton. In the new millennium, self-disclosure has become an equal opportunity activity used by millions of people, young and old, who blog daily, revealing a wide range of personal information to friends and strangers alike.

Finally, the Internet has brought about the most significant information revolution. Clients can often find, with the simple click of a mouse, an enormous amount of professional and personal information about their therapists, which may include hobbies, family members, political views, religious affiliation, even home address, and a quantity of other highly personal information. Internet directories also give clients a wide range of information about their therapists. Beyond the professional credentials and experience, such directories often provide photos of the therapists, which disclose age range and ethnicity among other things, and often also provide personal biographical information regarding hobbies and other interests. Consistent with consumer requests for information, more and more psychotherapists are constructing consumer-friendly, personal Web sites featuring not only professional data but also significant amounts of personal information. Blogs, chat rooms, or listservs with entries by therapists who identify themselves online are often accessible to the public and can result in extensive self-disclosure.

What the Therapy Setting Discloses

The psychotherapy office itself gives the client a wealth of information about the therapist. The therapist's office location, type of building, and type of neighboring offices or businesses give clients often significant first impressions. Another source of information is the office size, lighting, windows, view, and décor, which includes style of furniture, type of art displayed, personal mementos, books, religious symbols, and family photos. All these are personal self-disclosures that are not always as deliberate and intentional as verbal disclosures during sessions (Barnett, 1998; Gutheil & Gabbard, 1998; Mahalik, van Ormer, & Simi, 2000). Seating arrangements and spacing can be another form of self-disclosure. Whereas some therapists sit on a chair that is at the same level as the client's chair, others sit on a higher chair. Some sit behind a desk, others place a coffee table between themselves and the clients, and others leave a clear space.

Therapists who work out of their homes significantly increase the amount of self-disclosure of personal information. In the home office situation, the therapist reveals where he or she lives, the price range of the residence, what the neighborhood is like, and how well kept the homes, front lawns, and gardens are. Those who conduct sessions in the home itself rather than in a separate area also reveal how their living rooms are furnished and kept and even how clean the bathrooms are. Additionally, home office arrangements can disclose therapists' marital status, how many children they have, and even how well behaved the children are (for a detailed discussion of the home office, see chap. 7, this volume).

Therapists who practice in small or rural communities, on remote military bases, or in intimate and interconnected spiritual, ethnic, underprivileged, disabled, or college communities must all contend with extensive self-disclosure of their personal lives simply because many aspects are often displayed in clear view of their clients by virtue of the small community setting. In many of these small community situations, a therapist's marital status, family details, religion, political affiliation, sexual orientation, and other personal information may be readily available to clients (Brown, 1984; Campbell & Gordon, 2003; Hargrove, 1986; Nickel, 2004; Schank & Skovholt, 1997, 2006; Slattery, 2005; Stockman, 1990).

Client Considerations

Deliberate and intentional self-disclosure must be determined primarily by clients' needs and with sensitivity to clients' factors. Therapists must take into consideration how, for example, a family photo may have an impact on clients who struggle with intimate relationships or an expensive dress or ring may affect clients who struggle with financial matters.

Adult clients will generally have needs differing from younger clients. Indeed, children and other individuals who have a diminished capacity for abstract thought often benefit from more direct answers to questions requiring self-disclosure (Psychopathology Committee of the Group for the Advancement of Psychiatry, 2001). Because of the level of cognitive development, self-disclosure with this population may be the best way to establish a therapeutic alliance and trust. Adolescents are often resistant to therapy as they frequently see adult therapists as authority figures and extensions of their parents. Self-disclosure is one way to make adolescent clients feel honored and respected rather than judged and patronized.

Self-disclosure has a unique importance for therapists working with clients who hold particular religious or spiritual beliefs. These clients often ask therapists questions about their spiritual orientations and values as part of the interview process. Clients who are devout Christians, for example, often seem to work with therapists who share their spiritual beliefs whereas they are not likely to feel understood by atheist therapists. Additionally, many clients choose their therapists because they are aware of their spiritual orientation. These clients often meet their future therapists in the context of the church, synagogue, or meditation retreat (Geyer, 1994; Llewellyn, 2002; Montgomery & DeBell, 1997; Tillman, 1998).

Self-disclosure among gay male and lesbian clients is a very important issue as it relates to the key issue of being "out." Accordingly, several theorists agree that there is high therapeutic value in the therapists' self-disclosure of their sexual orientation (Isay, 1996; Mahalik et al., 2000; Tillman, 1998). Several studies have suggested that gay male and lesbian clients often prefer and seek therapists with the same sexual orientation, which apparently increases trust, affiliation, and therapeutic alliance (Bernstein, 2000; Goldstein, 1997; M. Jones, Botsko, & Gorman, 2003; Liddle, 1997; McDermott, Tyndall, & Lichtenberg, 1989). Unless the client already knows the therapist's sexual orientation prior to seeking therapy, very often the subject of their sexual orientation may be raised during the phone interview. As a result, self-disclosure is often a necessity for therapists who want to or choose to work with this population. Self-disclosure with gay male and lesbian clients has also been linked to the idea of a client's right to make informed decisions. On the basis of the assumption that psychotherapy is not value free and therapists have their own attitudes, values, and morals, gay male and lesbian clients have an understandable investment in ruling out therapists who practice "conversion therapy" or who otherwise do not value diverse sexual orientations before they even start therapy.

Similar to the concern of gay male and lesbian clients, studies of client–therapist similarity have revealed that clients from minority groups were often more comfortable with therapists who self-disclose or were observed or perceived by clients as coming from the same or a similar minority group. Such therapists were viewed as more trustworthy and expert than those from a dissimilar group (Sue & Sue, 2003). Therapists' self-disclosure has also been viewed as therapeutic in therapy groups treating war veterans with posttraumatic stress disorder, survivors of trauma, and women undergoing treatment for postabortion depression

(Barnett, 1998; Stricker & Fisher, 1990). Some therapists from the self-help tradition, or those who work primarily with gay male, lesbian, and other minority clients, take the position that self-disclosure leading to identification is essential for therapeutic success. Such an argument states that only war veteran therapists can fully empathize and successfully work with veteran clients, only gay male therapists should work with gay male clients, only lesbian therapists should work with lesbian clients, only women therapists can work successfully with women clients, and only Christian therapists can work with Christian clients. However, this assertion is not supported by research. It also does not seem practical, seeing as many male clients would be denied service in a field in which women therapists greatly outnumber male therapists.

Theoretical Orientations

Attitudes toward therapeutic self-disclosure, like the attitudes toward most other boundary crossings such as touch, gifts, or bartering, are closely related to the therapist's primary theoretical orientation. Yalom (1975) stated, "More than any other single characteristic, the nature and degree of therapist self-disclosure differentiates the various schools of . . . therapy" (p. 212). Generally, highly disclosing therapists view the focus of the psychotherapy process as an interconnection between the therapist and the client, whereas less disclosing therapists focus on working through clients' projections (C. Peterson, 2002; Stricker & Fisher, 1990).

Traditional analysts have followed Freud's instructions to serve as a mirror and a blank screen for the client, freeing the client to project her or his own feelings and thoughts on the neutral therapist. Neutrality and anonymity, according to traditional analytic theory, are the foundations for transference analysis. Despite Freud's own departure from these principles on occasion, most psychoanalysts and traditional psychodynamic psychotherapists adhere to general analytic neutrality and believe in the importance of minimizing self-disclosure for the purpose of achieving effective transference analysis (Langs, 1982; C. Peterson, 2002).

Self-disclosure is a way of responding to clients' questions, which, within the analytic tradition, is thought to result in gratification of clients' wishes rather than analysis of them (Mallow, 1998). Along these lines, Simon (1994) advocated that psychotherapists "Maintain therapist neutrality. Foster psychological separateness of the patient. . . . Preserve relative anonymity of the therapist" (p. 514). The last decade has seen a surge of willingness within the psychoanalytic–psychodynamic camp to explore the value of self-disclosure, in general, and more specifically, countertransference disclosure (e.g., Bridges, 2001; Cooper, 1998). Additionally, there is a growing acknowledgment that such things as tone of voice, body language, or office décor are all significant self-disclosures in psychoanalysis (Renik, 1996). The interpersonal focus of several modern psychodynamic psychotherapies has yielded an expanded body of knowledge illuminating the importance of self-disclosure in relational and intersubjective perspectives (Aron, 1991; Bridges, 2001; Burke, 1992; Cooper, 1998; Stricker & Fisher, 1990).

Humanistic and existential psychotherapies have emphasized the importance of self-disclosure in enhancing authentic therapeutic alliance, the most important factor in predicting clinical outcome (Lambert, 1991; Norcross & Goldfried, 1992). Humanistic practitioners assert that therapist self-disclosure makes clients feel more equal to, rather than inferior to, the therapists. It allows clients to recognize that all people have failings and unresolved matters in their lives and that there is no essential difference, in fact, between psychotherapists and clients (Stricker & Fisher, 1990; Williams, 1997). In discussing self-disclosure with clients, Bugental (1987) advocated, "First and foremost: strict honesty is required" (p. 143). Jourard (1971a), in his widely quoted book, *Self-Disclosure: An Experimental Analysis of the Transparent Self*, discussed at length the importance of self-disclosure for humanistic psychotherapy. He emphasized how self-disclosure enhances authentic relationships and increases therapeutic effectiveness because it encourages client honesty, frees the client to disclose difficult or shameful material, demystifies the therapist, deepens the dialogue between clients and therapists, and increases intimacy and satisfaction in the therapeutic process. Self-disclosure has been viewed as one of the most effective ways to enhance genuine encounters between therapists and clients and the most effective way to equalize the power differential so that intimate, mutual, and genuine relationships can be developed.

Group psychotherapy is another orientation that has stressed the importance of self-disclosure. Vinogradov and Yalom stated: "Group psychotherapists may—just like other members in the group—openly share their thoughts and feelings in a judicious and responsible manner, respond to others authentically and acknowledge or refute motives and feelings attributed to them" (1990, p. 198). Vinogradov and Yalom (1990) went on to encourage group therapists to reveal their feelings, to articulate the reasons for some of their behaviors, to acknowledge blind spots, and to demonstrate respect for the feedback offered by group members. Different modalities of group therapy, such as cognitive–behavioral, have relied on self-disclosure to promote positive therapeutic outcome.

Behavioral, cognitive, and cognitive–behavioral therapies have emphasized the importance of modeling, reinforcement, and normalizing in therapy and view self-disclosure as an effective vehicle to enhance these techniques (Freeman, Fleming, & Pretzer, 1990; Goldfried, Burckell, & Eubanks-Carter, 2003). In his best-selling book, *The Feeling Good Handbook,* Burns (1990) discussed the clinical effectiveness of honest feedback with certain clients. Similarly, Lazarus (1994), one of the founders of behavioral therapy, detailed the importance of therapists answering clients' appropriate questions. He further laid out the potential disruption to the clinical process that can result from therapists always responding to clients' questions with questions (e.g., "Can you tell me why you want to know?") rather than answering the questions. Fay (2002) described the effectiveness of helping clients reach a realistic assessment of their financial situation by sharing with his clients that, like them, he also lost a significant amount of money in the 2000 high-tech crash. In addition, on the basis of his assumption that clients feel less defective when they know the therapist can relate directly to the experience, he shared with clients who have paruresis (inhibited micturition in public bathrooms) that he himself had and overcame this problem. In similar fashion, several authors discuss the importance of self-disclosure in rational–emotive therapy. Modeling the rational–emotive process by using disclosures and examples from therapists' personal lives was reported to be a highly effective way to convince clients of its utility (Dryden, 1990; Tantillo, 2004).

Feminist therapy values therapists' self-disclosure for its role in fostering a more egalitarian relationship and solidarity between therapist and client, promoting clients' empowerment, and allowing them to make informed decisions in choosing female therapists as role models (Brown, 1994; Greenspan, 1986; Kessler & Waehler, 2005; Simi & Mahalik, 1997). The act of therapists and clients joining together in political demonstrations and other political activities is encouraged as a means to model and empower clients. Greenspan (1995) stated, "I am a great believer in the art of therapist self-disclosure as a way of deconstructing the isolation and shame that people experience in an individualistic and emotion-fearing culture" (p. 53).

Narrative therapy also places a high value on what they call therapists' transparency (White & Epston, 1990), and family therapy, Ericksonian therapy, and Adlerian therapy use it for the purposes of modeling and connection (Stricker & Fisher, 1990). The most common use of self-disclosure has been in the 12-step programs such as Alcoholics Anonymous, Over-Eaters Anonymous, and other self-help and peer-support models. As mentioned, many of these self-help modalities have entered the therapeutic mainstream and include clinician-facilitated support groups for addiction, parenting, abuse, rape, domestic violence, bereavement, or divorce. Self-disclosure by therapist–facilitators is essential for these programs (Mallow, 1998). Therapist–leaders' self-disclosure is even more powerful than that of other participants and is highly effective in reducing shame and guilt and provides a role model for the healing and recovery process.

The end of the 1990s and the beginning of the new millennium have also seen a significant increase in open discussion about flexible therapeutic boundaries, in general (e.g., Lazarus & Zur, 2002; Younggren & Gottlieb, 2004), and a surge in articles on self-disclosure, in particular (e.g., Bridges, 2001; C. Peterson, 2002). This includes a parallel focus on those settings for therapy in which self-disclosure is inevitable, for example, rural areas (Barnett, 1998; Simon & Williams, 1999), gay male and lesbian communities (Kessler & Waehler, 2005), and the military (Johnson, Ralph, &

Johnson, 2005). Similarly, the APA Ethics Code of 2002 introduced needed clarity to the issues when it provided a definition of "reasonable" that makes it clear that assessing the appropriateness of boundaries uses the "prevailing professional judgment of psychologists engaged in similar activities in similar circumstances" (p. 1061) rather than using only certain theoretical orientations or an arbitrary yardstick. Taken all together, it becomes clear that the professional attitudes toward self-disclosure have coevolved with the cultural attitudes toward self-disclosure (Williams, 1997; Zur, 2004b). Self-disclosure by therapists is no longer tied rigidly to theoretical orientation and has become an ever more acceptable therapeutic tool.

Self-Disclosure and Therapeutic Alliance

One of the main focuses of the research and writing on self-disclosure surrounds its relationship to the therapeutic alliance. Regardless of the therapeutic modality used, therapists' self-disclosure has been linked consistently to enhancement of therapeutic alliance, the best predictor of therapeutic outcome. Similarly, it has been reported to increase trust, familiarity, cooperation, intimacy, and reciprocal self-disclosure by clients (Barnett, 1998; Hanson, 2003; Knox et al., 1997). There is a sense that it creates more equality in the therapeutic relationship, which in turn facilitates a more open and trusting connection. It has been viewed as a form of gift-giving from therapist to client (Smolar, 2003) and a way to convey respect for the client as a mature collaborator in the therapeutic endeavor (Renik, 1996). Reports have also linked self-disclosure and the view of the therapist as a fellow human who is at times vulnerable. Furthermore, it seems to increase warmth, decrease anxiety, and model the clients' self-disclosure, as well as ways of handling and overcoming guilt and shame and demonstrating the therapist's willingness to take responsibility for a possible mistake. Self-disclosure that is in tune with clients' needs and personalities also reduces clients' sense of alienation and demonstrates the therapist's understanding of something the client is trying to convey (Bridges, 2001; Brown, 1994; Goldstein, 1997). Self-disclosure also must be done at the right time in the evolution of therapy. Sometimes premature self-disclosure may be overwhelming or unwelcome by the client. Similarly, a belated self-disclosure may lead to a sense of betrayal and rouse distrust, as is the case when a client finds out after the fact that his or her therapist went through a major operation, had a child, or got married.

Case Study: Too Much Information

A middle-age female therapist was working in a wealthy suburb of a major city with a 40-year-old, reserved, upper-class woman of northern European ancestry who presented with postpartum depression. This client insisted on addressing the therapist as "Doctor" and made it clear that she was to be addressed formally as Mrs. Jones. The woman was ashamed of not being able to enjoy her newborn baby and felt guilty about being "such a bad mother." She also claimed to be worried lest the baby be negatively affected by her indifference. She seemed to feel also that there were deep, complex echoes from her own infancy and childhood that the therapist could unravel and free her of her distress.

The therapist, who came from a more liberal and open tradition, was willing to disclose personal information if and when it might be helpful. Yet she was aware that at this point revealing to the woman that she, the therapist, had also had postpartum depression might not be a very effective clinical intervention. It might very well interfere with the early stage of treatment and appear unprofessional to the client who held a very conventional, stereotypic image of the "Doctor." The client saw the therapist exclusively in her authority role and not necessarily as a woman who might be a mother, too. The client refused the therapist's suggestion for a medication evaluation with a psychiatrist because she was ashamed of her depression and was concerned that the medication might interfere with nursing or adversely affect the baby.

As the treatment was not progressing, the therapist considered her options with full appreciation that this upper-class client was not very affiliative. The therapist was aware that thus far the client's culture and style determined the rather professionally cold tenor of therapy. She believed that after this first phase, during which they established the basic therapeutic relationship, she might then be able to clinically use that she is also a mother who had postpartum depression. The therapist elected to introduce the fact that she is a mother through a nonintrusive self-disclosure by placing a picture of her 1-year-old daughter on her desk in her office. The rationale was that such an action is consistent with the client's culture and expectations and would not likely to be perceived as unprofessional by the client.

Timing indeed proved to be the crucial element that created an opportunity for effective self-disclosure. A few sessions later, the client mentioned the photo and asked if the girl in the photo was the therapist's daughter. This, obviously, gave the therapist the opportunity to reveal more details about her baby girl. In subsequent sessions, the client continued to refer to the photo and after waiting for the opportune moment, the therapist disclosed that she, too, had postpartum depression. By then, the client was ready to hear the information. The disclosure that the therapist also had postpartum depression was designed to make the client more hopeful that she could also overcome her depression while simultaneously removing the shame and stigma of personal failure that the client associated with it. In summary, sensitive consideration of client factors, stages in the evolution of therapeutic alliance, and therapist factors led to successful strategic clinical use of the therapist's self-disclosure.

10

Touch in Therapy

Touch in therapy has probably been the most controversial of all boundary crossings because of the cultural and professional associations of touch with sexuality. The major concern is that nonsexual touch may lead to sexual touch and sexual exploitation. As a result, touch has become a major risk management concern. Gutheil and Gabbard (1993) stated that from a risk management point of view, "a handshake is about the limit of social physical contact" (p. 195).

The conflict around the use of touch in therapy arises from a number of sources. There is tension between, on the one side, well-established scientific knowledge that says that touch is important for human development and, on the other side, the ethical concerns with exploitative and harmful sexual touching of clients by therapists. A vast amount of scientific data has been acquired in the past half century on the importance of touch for bonding, human development, healing, and communication (Bowlby, 1969; Field, 1998; Harlow, 1971; Montagu, 1971). The clinical utility of touch in therapy has also been studied extensively and has determined conclusively that touch enhances therapeutic alliance and increases a sense of trust, calm, and safety (e.g., Hunter & Struve, 1998; E. Smith, Clance, & Imes, 1998). However, there is a major concern that nonsexual touch may lead to sexual touch and exploitation of clients (Bersoff, 1999; Gabbard, 1989; Pope & Vasquez, 2001; Rutter, 1989; Simon, 1991, 1994). Paradoxically, most psychotherapists' surveys reveal that 87% of therapists touch their clients (Tirnauer, Smith, & Foster, 1996), 85% hug their clients (Pope, Tabachnick, & Keith-Spiegel, 1987), and 65% approve of touch as an adjunct to verbal psychotherapy (Schultz, 1975). It seems, in spite of the risk management viewpoint that touch is taboo, most therapists do touch their clients, and do so appropriately.

Like almost all interventions and boundary crossings, the meaning of touch can only be understood in relation to the client factors, therapeutic setting, therapeutic orientation, therapeutic relationship, and therapist factors. Touch, when viewed through the prism of these factors, can have radically different contextual meanings (Hedges, Hilton, Hilton, & Caudill, 1997; Koocher & Keith-Spiegel, 1998; E. Smith et al., 1998).

This chapter discusses the issues of touch as an adjunct to verbal psychotherapy and reviews the literature on body psychotherapies in which touch is often the primary therapeutic tool. Touch, here, refers primarily to physical contact initiated by the therapist. However, even when a client initiates a handshake or a hug, it is the therapists' responsibility to use their clinical judgment, in each therapeutic situation, to ascertain whether responding positively to the clients' wish to touch is ethical and clinically advantageous.

Touch as an Ethical and Boundary Issue

The relationship among boundaries, touch, and psychotherapy presents a unique situation that involves three main types of boundaries. The first is the distinct boundary of the physical body, the second is concerned with psychotherapeutic boundaries, and the third relates to the boundary between sexual and nonsexual touch. The boundary of the body is clear and well defined by the skin. Although the skin is physically, distinctly defined and separates individuals from their environment, it is also a gateway for numerous complex and often mysterious physiological and emotional regulatory systems that are affected when the skin is touched.

Touch between therapists and clients represents one of the most recognized psychotherapeutic boundaries, as it reaches across the traditional professional–interpersonal space separating therapists and clients. Harmful boundary violations occur when therapists engage in sexual relationships with clients. In contrast to sexual boundary violations, a client-initiated handshake at the beginning or end of a session, an appropriate and encouraging pat on the client's back, supportive hand-holding, or a nonsexual hug can be exceedingly helpful, clinical boundary crossings. Additionally, specially trained body psychotherapists, such as Reichian or bioenergetics therapists, who use thoroughly researched and established hands-on techniques, are also engaged in therapeutic boundary crossing.

Some differentiations between sexual and nonsexual touch in therapy focus on the areas touched (i.e., hand vs. genitals), others focus on whether the intent is to sexually arouse the client or the therapist, and yet others propose an encompassing view that "erotic touch" is any behavior that leads to sexual arousal (e.g., Brodsky, 1985; Pope, Sonne, & Holroyd, 1993). Help with differentiation between sexual and nonsexual touch in therapy comes from one of the key studies that found correlations between nonsexual touch and sexual touch. The study showed that the sexual boundary violation was positively correlated, not with touch per se, but with the frequency that therapists touched clients of the opposite sex in comparison with the frequency of touch of clients of the same sex (Holroyd & Brodsky, 1980). The important conclusion of the findings was that therapists' own attitudes toward touch and whether they tend to generally sexualize all forms of touch is the determining factor in whether they are likely to blur sexual and nonsexual forms of touch.

The debate about touch in therapy started with the inception of the new profession early in the 20th century. Ferenczi, originally trained in the psychoanalytic model, at one point spoke out as a proponent of nonerotic hugging, holding, and kissing of clients, believing that the use of such therapeutic touch would provide corrective parenting to clients with early injuries. As mentioned previously, Freud was supportive initially, but withdrew his support when he became aware that Ferenczi had become sexually and romantically involved with more than one of his clients. He wished to protect the budding psychoanalytic method from falling into disrepute. Ferenczi refused to stop touching his clients altogether and was subsequently expelled from the ranks of orthodox psychoanalysis (Fosshage, 2000). Wilhelm Reich (1972), who developed the most comprehensive method of clinical touch, was, like Ferenczi, one of Freud's inner circle and prominent in the International Psychoanalytic Association. He, too, was ousted from the International Psychoanalytic Association for his professional stance on touch in therapy.

Since that time, regardless of the extensive scientific data accumulated on the importance of touch for human development, for healing in general and specifically in psychotherapy, the field of psychotherapy has generally shied away from discussing touch as a clinical intervention and instead has discussed it as an ethical and risk management concern. The ambivalence regarding touch was initiated by the psychoanalytical concern with the impact of touch on the therapeutic frame and transference analysis. The other source of concern has focused on the power differential and the potential for sexual exploitation of clients by their therapists. Since the early 1990s, the primary concern has shifted even further to the concern that even casual touch might lead to therapists going down the slippery slope into sexual boundary violations (Gabbard, 1989; Gutheil & Gabbard, 1993; Pope & Vasquez, 2001; Strasburger, Jorgenson, & Sutherland, 1992). Sexualizing therapeutic touch and most other forms of touch reflect modern, Western, cultural beliefs in which relationships among sensuality, physical sensation, and sexuality are intertwined (Dineen, 1996; Zur, 2004b). Part of the problem with differentiating sexual and nonsexual touch in therapy stems from the lack of differentiation between sexual feeling and sexual activity. Although about 90% of therapists report being sexually attracted to their clients at some time, fewer than 10% have ever consummated a sexual relationship with their clients (Pope et al., 1993; Pope & Vasquez, 2001). Pope et al. (1987), prominent researchers on therapists' ethical attitudes and behavior, reflected on the carryover between risk management concerns and the legitimate utility of touch in therapy. They stated, "The focus on erotic contact in therapy has raised questions about the legitimacy and effects of ostensibly non-erotic physical contact" (p. 1001). Similarly, Holroyd and Brodsky (1980) titled their article regarding their survey, "Does touching clients lead to sexual intercourse?" Not surprisingly, they also concluded that it "is difficult to determine where 'non-erotic hugging, kissing, and affectionate touching' leave off and 'erotic contact' begins" (p. 810).

Ethics and Standard of Care Considerations

Nonsexual, clinically appropriate touch in psychotherapy is neither unethical nor below the standard of care. Like the APA Ethics Code (American Psychological Association, 2002), ethics codes of all major psychotherapy professional associations (e.g., American Association for Marriage and Family Therapists, 2001; American Counseling Association, 2005; National Association of Social Workers, 1999) do not prohibit the use of appropriate touch in therapy (see Appendix B, this volume, for details). All psychotherapy professional codes of ethics view sexual or violent touch with a current client as unethical. As with any clinical intervention, touch should be used ethically with the client's welfare in mind, taking into consideration the client's many personal factors. For obvious reasons, the ethics of touch receive the most extensive coverage in the Ethical Guidelines of the U.S. Association of Body Psychotherapy (2001), which clearly articulates the ethical guidelines for the use of touch in therapy, the importance of informed consent, and concerns with respect, diversity, consultation, record keeping, treatment plans, and many other pertinent issues for ethical touch in psychotherapy.

Most body psychotherapists, who have a number of clinical orientations, such as Reichian (Reich, 1972) or bioenergetics (Lowen, 1976), use actual touch as their primary tool in psychotherapy. The introduction to the U.S. Association of Body Psychotherapy (2001) Ethical Guidelines states,

> Body psychotherapists recognize the intrinsic unity of the human being in our somatic nature. Body psychotherapists, therefore, work in ways that foster the integration of bodily sensation, thought, affect, and movement to promote more integral human functioning and the resolution of psychotherapeutic concerns. Body psychotherapeutic methods, including language, gesture and touch, when used in responsible, ethical and competent ways, make an essential contribution to the psychotherapeutic process by including the missing and

often alienated aspects of our being which are rooted in our bodily nature and experience. (Introduction, para. 2)

Body psychotherapists view the body–mind as a feedback loop or continuum rather than two separate systems. They believe that any event has holistic impact, involving physical, cognitive, spiritual, and emotional elements. Healthy functioning and dysfunction in any part of the organisms' continuum will affect the whole system (Field, 1998; E. Smith et al., 1998). Wilhelm Reich (1972), the originator of Reichian therapy, is often referred to as the grandfather of body-oriented psychotherapy. He worked to dismantle the barriers and restrictions to touch that had been imposed by the dominant influences of early psychoanalysis. Body psychotherapy assists people to heal and develop, not only through the use of verbal, cognitive, affective, or behavioral interventions, but also by guiding them to a deeper awareness of their bodily sensations, images, behavior, and feelings. Techniques common to most body-centered psychotherapies include attention to somatic awareness, breath, movement, and imagery. The forms of touch may vary from deep manipulation, used to release body blocks, to supportive hugs or holding. Beside Reich and bioenergetics (Lowen, 1976), other forms of body psychotherapy include Hakomi therapy, Gay and Kathy Hendricks's radiance method, Amy and Arnold Mindells's process therapy, Christine Caldwell's moving cycle, and the Rubenfeld synergy system (Nordmarken & Zur, 2004).

Types of Touch in Therapy

Touch, in the context of this section, refers to any physical contact occurring between therapists and clients. Therapists can deliberately use many forms of touch as an adjunct to verbal psychotherapy. These forms of touch are intentionally and strategically used to enhance a sense of connection with the client and to soothe, greet, relax, or reassure the client. Their use is also intended to reduce anxiety, slow heartbeat, physically and emotionally calm the client, or assist the client in moving out of a dissociative state. Therapeutic touch, in this context, most often includes a hug, light touch, hand-holding, or rubbing a client's back, shoulder, or arm. Based partly on formulations by Downey (2001), Nordmarken and Zur (2004), and E. Smith et al. (1998), the following are descriptions of touch in therapy that is used as an adjunct to verbal psychotherapy, touch as the main tool in body psychotherapy, and inappropriate–unethical touch.

☐ *Ritualistic or socially accepted gestures for greeting and goodbye or arrival and departure:* These gestures figure significantly among most cultures and include handshakes, a greeting, or farewell embrace, and other culturally accepted gestures.

☐ *Conversational marker:* This form of light touch on the arm, hand, back, or shoulder is intended to make or highlight a point and can also take place at times of stillness, with the purpose of accentuating the therapist's presence and conveying attention.

☐ *Consolatory touch:* This important form of touch, holding the hands or shoulders of a client or providing a comforting hug, is most likely to enhance therapeutic alliance.

☐ *Reassuring touch:* This form of touch is geared to encouraging and reassuring clients and usually involves a pat on the back or shoulder.

☐ *Playful touch:* This form of touch, mostly of hand, shoulders, or head, may take place while playing a game with a child or adolescent client.

☐ *Grounding or reorienting touch:* This form of touch is intended to help clients reduce anxiety or dissociation by using touch to the hand or arm or by leading them to touch their own hands or arms.

☐ *Task-oriented touch:* This involves touch that is merely ancillary to the task at hand, such as offering a hand to help someone stand up or bracing an arm around a client's shoulders to keep the client from falling.

☐ *Corrective experience:* This form of touch may involve the holding of an adult or rocking of a child by a therapist who practices forms of therapy that emphasize the importance of corrective experiences.

☐ *Instructional or modeling touch:* Therapists may model how to touch or respond to touch by demonstrating a firm handshake, holding an agitated child, or responding to unwanted touch.

☐ *Celebratory or congratulatory touch:* The therapist may give a pat on the back or a congratulatory hug to a client who has achieved a goal.

☐ *Experiential touch:* This form of touch usually takes place when the therapist conducts an experiential exercise, such as teaching gestures during assertiveness training, or in family sculpturing in which family members are asked to assume certain positions in relationship to each other.

☐ *Referential touch:* This is often done in group or family therapy when the therapist lightly taps the arm or shoulder of a client, indicating that he or she can take a turn or be silent.

☐ *Inadvertent touch:* This is touch that is unintentional, involuntary, and unpremeditated, such as an inadvertent brush against a client by the therapist.

☐ *Touch intended to prevent a client from hurting him- or herself:* This type of touch is intended to stop self-harming behaviors such as head banging, self-hitting, or self-cutting.

☐ *Touch intended to prevent someone from hurting another:* This form of touch is intended to stop or restrain someone from hurting another person, as sometimes happens in family, couple, or group therapy or when working with extremely volatile clients.

☐ *Touch in therapists' self-defense:* This form of touch is used by a therapist to physically defend himself or herself from the assault of a violent client by using self-defense techniques that restrain clients with minimum force.

☐ *Therapeutic touch in body psychotherapies:* This is different from the use of touch as an adjunct to verbal psychotherapy. Somatic and body psychotherapists regularly use touch as part of their theoretically prescribed clinical intervention. Massage, Rolfing, or other hands-on techniques incorporated or implemented consecutively with psychotherapy also fit into this category.

In contrast to the aforementioned forms of touch, there are also inappropriate forms of touch. The following three forms of touch in psychotherapy are unethical and, depending on the state, often illegal. They are counterclinical and should always be avoided.

☐ *Sexual touch:* The initiator of this form of touch, between therapist and a current client, intends to sexually arouse

the therapist, the client, or both. This is always unethical
and counterclinical. It is illegal in many states. Even when
a client initiates the sexual touch, it is still the therapist's
responsibility to stop it.
☐ *Hostile–violent touch:* It is always highly inappropriate and
unethical for a therapist to touch a client in a physically
hostile or violent manner.
☐ *Punishing touch:* Physical punishment, by a therapist, is
never appropriate in the context of psychotherapy.

Scientific and Cultural Views on Touch

Let us now look at touch in the context of the scientific evaluation
of what Montagu (1971) called the "mother of all senses," with an
additional focus on how touch is viewed in many societies, principally in the United States. Language never completely super-
sedes the more primitive forms of communication such as tone of
voice and physical touch (Frank, 1973). Recent discoveries in neu-
roscience provide us with a picture of the importance of nonverbal communication. From paleocircuits in the spinal cord, brain
stem, basal ganglia, and limbic system, nonverbal cues are pro-
duced and received below the level of conscious awareness.
Hence, memories engendered by nonverbal communication remain with us long after words have died away (M. Knapp & Hall,
1997). Individuals vary with regard to the mode of nonverbal communication they primarily rely on, whether it is auditory, visual,
olfactory, or tactile.

Freud identified the first year of life as the oral stage and, for
decades, it was believed that babies bonded with caregivers simply because they fed them. Although attachment and bonding
imply intimate touch, it was not until the 1950s that the link between parent–child touch and attachment became clear. Following World War II, psychologists explored children's responses to
separation and how parenting styles affected the quality of attachment. They concluded that bonding occurred not only in response to the reduction of primary drives but also to "primary
object clinging," ergo a need for intimate contact (Ainsworth, 1978;
Bowlby, 1969).

In the 1950s, Harlow (1971) conducted his breakthrough experiments demonstrating the importance of touch for bonding and healthy development through his controlled laboratory research on infant monkeys. He discovered that "comfort contact" proved to be a more significant parenting quality than feeding and that touch, not food, bound infant to caregiver. His studies also revealed that at least one half hour per day of interactive touch was needed to support normal development and that monkeys deprived of interactive touch became neurotic and asocial and exhibited various abnormal behaviors as adults. Harlow's studies supported what had been discovered about the needs of human infants as well. The absence of loving touch had been documented to have a profound impact on the will to live, and when the need for human touch remained unsatisfied, abnormal behavior resulted (Montagu, 1971). Death rates for undertouched infants in institutes during the 1920s ranged from 30% to 100% (Hunter & Struve, 1998). Children who were undertouched tended to have great difficulty feeling of value, feeling truly powerful, or forming reciprocally supportive relationships as adults (Heller, 1997).

Montagu (1971) identified touch as humans' first language. Long before infants can see an image, smell an odor, taste a flavor, or hear a sound, they experience themselves and others through touch, their only reciprocal sense. Touch is, indeed, the first sense to develop in the embryo, and all other senses—sight, sound, taste, and smell—are derived from it. Loving touch in the early years is essential to adequate neurological and emotional development (Bowlby, 1969; Harlow, 1971). Studies in bonding also showed that human babies who were held often and touched frequently in their earliest stages of development had higher scores on physical, emotional, and interpersonal scales (Field, 1998). The tactile system is the earliest sensory system to become functional in the embryo, and there are indications that it may be the last to fade (Fosshage, 2000). It remains a potent form of communication throughout the course of one's life.

Whereas many of the physiological ramifications of touch are universal, the interpersonal meaning of touch can only be understood in its sociocultural context. Researchers have organized cultural attitudes toward touch on a continuum of tactility whereby people of Germanic origin are found to be least tactile, Americans and English are only slightly higher, Scandinavians occupy the middle position, and those of Latin and Mediterranean place at the high end (Jourard, 1971b; Mehrabian, 1971). Asians, depending on the country, lie anywhere from low to high on the continuum.

North Americans, in general, are wary of touch, although within the culture there are differences regarding touch between different regions, classes, and ethnic or minority groups, which align well with the continuum mentioned previously. Research on touch revealed that many unspoken protocols continued to inhibit touch between classes and racially or ethnically diverse groups, for example, between Caucasians and African Americans in the late 1990s in America, and little has changed since then (Hunter & Struve, 1998). Euro-American cultures, in general, and particularly that of North American White, Anglo-Saxon Protestants, have developed a set of unspoken taboos or rules regarding touch. These taboos or rules include "Don't touch the opposite sex!" "Don't touch yourself!" "Don't touch strangers!" "Do not touch the elderly, the sick, and the dying!" and "Do not touch those who are of higher status!" (Cohen, 1987; E. Smith et al., 1998).

Attitudes toward touch are also demonstrated in the child-rearing practices of various cultures. American babies and children are among the least touched in comparison with other cultures (Heller, 1997). The high value given to early independence and self-sufficiency has resulted in American parents distancing themselves physically from their children. The largest percentage of insecure children are found in cultures, such as the United States, that do not value touch and require the earliest self-reliance, whereas those cultures that touch more and value interdependence have the highest percentage of securely attached infants (M. E. Lamb, Thompson, Gardner, & Charnov, 1985). A review of 49 societies concluded that a lack of bodily pleasure derived from touching and stroking during the formative periods of life was significantly associated with violent behavior in adults (Prescott, 1975).

In American culture, there is often a propensity to infantilize or sexualize physical contact or to link it with aggression. That means that touch is, primarily, culturally reserved for children or sexual or aggressive contacts. As a result, Americans tend to avoid touch for fear of being misunderstood (Hunter & Struve, 1998). Children are touched more frequently and most comfortably compared with adults, whereas most public displays of affection between adults are held suspect. This is especially true of men touching men, who are, however, allowed to touch in competitive sports and in military action. As far as sexualization of innocent touch is concerned, the restrictive idea that sensual pleasures were sinful was embedded in American culture first through the Puritanism of the Pilgrims and amplified with the arrival of the Victorian era (Dineen, 1996). It survives, albeit in a muted form, even today. This fear that affectionate touch might be sexually motivated or might "slip" into sexual touch is the legacy of earlier generations and seems destined to permeate the attitudes regarding touch in American culture into the future. The high rate of sexual abuse in our culture and the more recent exposure of sexual abuse by priests have added even further to the hesitation to touch children.

Touch in Context

Touch, when viewed through the prism of client factors, therapeutic setting, therapeutic orientation, therapeutic relationship, and therapist factors, can have radically different contextual meanings (Hedges et al., 1997; Koocher & Keith-Spiegel, 1998; E. Smith et al., 1998).

Client factors, which include age, gender, presenting problem, diagnosis, personality, personal touch history, culture, and class, are highly relevant to the meaning and potential healing effect of touch in therapy. What is particularly appropriate and effective with one client may be inappropriate and even damaging with another. Letting a young child jump into the therapist's lap may be very appropriate, but it is not permissible with an adult client. Reaching out gently and respectfully to hold the hand of a grieving mother may not have the intended positive effect if the same is done in early stages of therapy with a survivor of sexual abuse. In large part, clients' individual experiences and relationships to touch are of the utmost importance. Elements of personal space are defined within a culture and affect the interpretation of therapeutic touch. In this context, a therapist's touch, or lack of touch, may be seen as distant, respectful, or invasive depending on the socialization and experience of the individual client (E. Smith et al., 1998). Although there is a growing body of literature on multicultural theory and counseling (Aponte & Wohl, 2000; Sue & Sue, 2003), relatively little has been written specifically on the use of touch in psychotherapy with ethnically diverse populations.

Gender issues are also extremely important in understanding the context of touch, and the clients' personal experience and relationship to being touched by someone of the same gender or opposite gender affect the response. Touch in psychotherapy occurs between therapists of both sexes and their female and male clients as well as same-sex therapist–client dyads (Brodsky, 1985). As noted earlier, any clinical intervention, such as touch, that is reserved for only one sex may be interpreted as being potentially sexist and increasing the probability of boundary violation (Holroyd & Brodsky, 1980). Research has confirmed that women respond more positively to touch than do men (Hunter & Struve, 1998). From birth, American females receive more affectionate touch from males and females and are given greater permission to touch either gender and be touched by either gender. They are more likely to have and expect a broader repertoire of touch, and they are less likely than men to perceive sexual intent in men when touched by them (Downey, 2001). In contrast, American males are given less affectionate touch in infancy and early childhood, and this has been linked with higher rates of violence and aggression in later life. Therefore, they may lack a wide repertoire of touch and are more likely to sexualize touch that is not hostile or aggressive. They are also likely to perceive sexual intent when women touch them, especially when the situation is ambiguous or casual (E. Smith et al., 1998).

The use of touch with survivors of childhood trauma has been much debated. Whereas some authors assert that touch in any form should never be used with this population, many others agree that the clinically appropriate and ethical use of touch with survivors of childhood abuse, when applied cautiously, can be invaluable in helping them heal and recover from their traumatic experiences. The concern is that there is a possibility that touch used with these clients may recreate, evoke, or retraumatize previous client-experienced dynamics of victimization (Lawry, 1998). Cornell (1997) stated that once a strong therapeutic alliance has been formed, "the use of touch will evoke, address and hopefully help correct such historical experiences and distortion" (p. 33). What seems to be of the highest importance is that the client must want to be touched and understand the concepts of choice and personal empowerment before it is clinically or ethically appropriate to begin the use of touch in session. To this end, clients should be encouraged to express their preferences, to practice boundary-setting exercises, and to participate in creating a treatment plan. Studies suggest that there is a positive correlation between a client's perception that they are in control of touch and their positive evaluation of touch in psychotherapy. Research has also found that sexually abused clients were more likely to attribute a corrective or educative role to touch in therapy than were nonabused clients. Of these clients, 71% reported that touch repaired self-esteem, trust, and a sense of their own power or agency, especially in setting limits and asking for what they need (E. Smith et al., 1998).

Consistent with the pattern in the general culture, therapists tend to touch young clients more often than they do their adult clients, and female therapists touch child clients more often than male therapists do (Hunter & Struve, 1998). A growing body of literature has linked aggressive, violent, and antisocial behaviors to early childhood touch deprivation (Field, 1998; Montagu, 1971; Older, 1982). Touch-deprived children often grow up with a diminished ability to identify and experience emotions, in general, and a reduced ability to initiate or receive touch (Hunter & Struve, 1998). Research has demonstrated that when the staff of an adolescent treatment program modeled nonsexual, nonviolent touch and incorporated physical contact as an acceptable aspect of the milieu, the adolescents demonstrated a marked decrease in violent and sexual behaviors (Dunne, Bruggen, & O'Brien, 1982). Touch is usually contraindicated for clients who are actively paranoid, hostile, or aggressive or who implicitly or explicitly demand touch (Durana, 1998).

Most people experience some diminution in physical faculties and perceptual skills as they age, but the sense of touch generally remains intact and is valued as increasingly important as a source of contact and communication. The soothing, affirming experience of touch is most important at the beginning and end of one's life and generous, nurturing touch can gently facilitate the process of aging and dying with dignity (Hollinger, 1986).

The setting of therapy is profoundly important in evaluating the efficacy and meaning of touch. Some settings, such as prisons, are likely to restrict touch, whereas children or hospice clinics are likely to encourage it. Obviously, practicing in different cultural milieus is likely to result in different attitudes and use of touch. Latino or Middle Eastern clients are likely to endorse and expect physical touch more than Northern European, Japanese, or North American clients (E. Smith et al., 1998). Ethnicity, gender, and class also have direct implications for touch in psychotherapy, as touch has layers of meaning depending on one's culture, socialization, and individual experience. With levels of class and authority, it often moves from higher to lower; that is, a higher ranking individual may initiate touch of a subordinate but not vice versa. The same is true of male-to-female interaction in some societies (Halbrook & Duplechin, 1994).

Therapeutic relationships or the nature of the therapeutic alliance is one of the most important factors determining the potential efficacy of the use of touch in therapy. Therapist–client relationships of trust and of long duration are likely to create a familiar and safe context for effective use of touch in therapy. In contrast, short or conflicting relationships are less likely to be conducive to it. The relationships between touch and the therapeutic alliance seem to be bidirectional. As reported earlier, appropriate and "intune" touch significantly enhanced positive therapeutic alliance (Horton, Clance, Sterk-Elifson, & Emshoff, 1995; E. Smith et al., 1998) and, in return, created a further atmosphere of trust and the possibility of the further use of clinically appropriate touch.

As with all other boundary considerations, therapeutic orientation is exceptionally relevant in the clinical usefulness of touch in therapy. Body psychotherapists' clinical orientations, such as Reichian (Reich, 1972) or bioenergetics (Lowen, 1976), often use touch as their primary tool in psychotherapy. In contrast, most traditional psychoanalysts are generally opposed to any form of touch in therapy (Menninger, 1958; E. Smith et al., 1988; Wolberg, 1967). However, many other orientations support the clinically appropriate use of touch (Milakovitch, 1993; Williams, 1997). A few modern analysts, such as Fosshage (2000), have differed with mainstream analytic doctrine and advocate a clinically responsible use of touch in psychoanalysis.

The human potential movement and the humanistic movement of the 1960s introduced a whole new approach to touch and boundaries in therapy. This movement endorsed appropriate nonerotic touch and viewed it as an enhancement of the therapist–client connection (Hunter & Struve, 1998). Rogers (1970) discussed the value of touch and described specifically how he soothed clients by holding, embracing, and kissing them. Gestalt therapy incorporates numerous forms of touch as an integral part of therapy (Perls, 1973). Gestalt practitioners place a special importance on nonverbal communication and nonverbal intervention. Unfortunately, gestalt practices in the 1960s and early 1970s, under Perls's leadership, went too far and at times included unethical sexual touch in conjunction with therapy (Hunter & Struve, 1998). Family therapists, including Satir (1972), often use touch as an element of engaging clients in therapy (Holub & Lee, 1990). Behavioral and cognitive–behavioral therapists are likely to incorporate touch or any boundary crossing into therapy if it fits with their interventions such as modeling or reinforcement (Lazarus & Zur, 2002).

In their survey of therapists, Pope et al. (1987) reported that therapists of differing theoretical orientations have very different beliefs about the effect and practice of touching clients. They reported that 30% of humanistic therapists indicated that nonerotic hugging, kissing, and affectionate touching might frequently benefit clients in psychotherapy. In contrast, only 6% of psychodynamic therapists indicated the same. Whereas most psychodynamic therapists thought touch could be easily misunderstood, humanistic therapists did not share this view. Similarly, Milakovitch (1993) compared therapists who use or do not use touch and reported that therapists who use touch are likely to subscribe to a humanistic theoretical orientation, whereas therapists who do not use touch usually subscribe to a psychodynamic orientation.

Therapists' culture, age, and professional socializations are likely to affect their utilization of clinical touch. Older therapists were socialized to practice with less fear of boundary crossing (Williams, 1997) and are more likely to use touch more casually than younger ones whose training included much more focus on risk management and defensive medicine. Therapists' own culture is very likely to determine their personal comfort with touch and, therefore, its use in the clinical settings. Milakovitch (1993) compared therapists who touch and those who do not touch and found that beside the therapeutic orientation factor, therapists who touch obviously value touch in therapy and believe that gratifying the need to be touched is important. Therapists who do not touch believe that gratifying the need to be touched is detrimental to therapy and the client. Unlike therapists who do not touch, therapists who touch were more likely to be touched by their own therapists and had supervisors and professors who believe in the legitimacy of touch as a therapeutic tool. Therapists who touch were more likely to experience body psychotherapies than therapists who do not touch. In contrast to therapists who do not touch, therapists who touch are more supportive of models that use touch and body psychotherapy techniques. Female therapists tend to touch their clients more often than do male therapists. Pope and Vasquez (2001) articulated their assessment of therapists' use of touch in therapy:

> If the therapist is personally comfortable engaging in physical contact with a patient, maintains a theoretical orientation for which therapist–client contact is not antithetical, and has competence (education, training and supervised experience) in the use of touch, then the decision of whether or not to make physical contact with a particular client must be based on a careful evaluation of the clinical needs of the client at that moment. When solidly based upon clinical needs and a clinical rationale, touch can be exceptionally caring, comforting, reassuring, or healing. (p. 170)

Case Study: A Touchy Subject

A 30-year-old Caucasian woman was seeing a middle-aged, male therapist. She presented with anxiety and described a history of having been molested as a child. She quickly became emotionally dependent on the therapist, whom she found caring, smart, and attractive. After several months in therapy, she started processing her molestation experience, which triggered general anxiety and frequent bouts of weeping. During these times of distress, she asked if he would hold her hands.

The therapist was aware that using touch with those who have experienced a sexual boundary violation can be a very sensitive matter indeed, requiring the utmost caution. He knew he had to consider a number of relevant factors. Appropriately, he first considered the gender difference between him and the client, her attraction to him, and the fact that his practice was very private and involved neither a receptionist nor a next-door colleague. Being a conscientious therapist, he checked his feelings to ascertain that although he liked her, he was not attracted to her in a romantic or sexual way. He also considered the vast amount of research confirming the general clinical utility of touch. More specifically, he considered the research indicating that appropriate, consensual, and respectful touch with clients traumatized in childhood was reported to be clinically effective in restoring clients' self-esteem, trust, and a sense of power in setting limits.

After following the step-by-step risk–benefit evaluation, he felt intuitively that responding to her and touching her hand would, most likely, enhance the therapeutic alliance and he knew that that alliance is the best predictor of positive therapeutic outcome. Yet he was unwilling to rely solely on a gut feeling.

There was always the possibility that holding her hand might be interpreted as a sexual gesture or, most seriously, might trigger dynamics of submission and victimization, entrapment, anger, fear, vulnerability, and feelings of worthlessness. Either could be highly disruptive to the therapeutic process and harming to the client. Additionally, even if he refused gently, she could easily perceive it as a rejection. This might trigger a shame response as well, which in turn would be likely to exacerbate her anxiety. There was also the possibility that not responding to her wish to have her hand held but continuing to "hold" her emotionally might support the notion that therapy is safe and boundaries are not being crossed lightly.

Recognizing that the ethical decision-making process had not resulted in a clear or obvious conclusion, the therapist sought a consultation with a former supervisor who was an expert on working with trauma victims and the ethical use of touch in therapy. Through consultation, the therapist realized that rather than making his own decision and risking therapeutic rupture, he could bring the question and his quandary to the next session and engage the client in a discussion of the issues of touch and boundaries and detailing his concerns. Thus he would also model to her how to exercise control over her own emotional, physical, and sexual boundaries. As a prudent therapist, he detailed his ethical and clinical considerations in the clinical records.

11

Gifts

G iving a gift is an ancient and universal way to express, among other things, gratitude, appreciation, altruism, and love. Most often, a gift is considered something that is bestowed voluntarily and without compensation. Psychologists, sociologists, and anthropologists who have studied gift-giving behavior view it as a product of an interaction between psychological mechanisms, such as altruism or a wish to reward, and environmental–cultural customs, values, and mores (Saad & Gill, 2003). Most commonly, clients give gifts to therapists; therapists sometimes give gifts to their clients; and related nonclient third parties, such as parents of a child–client, may give gifts to therapists. The appropriateness and the meaning of clients' gifts, how to respond to them, and whether to interpret or accept them have been the focus of discussions in the field of psychotherapy around the issue gift-giving.

There are several types and forms of gifts in psychotherapy. Gifts can be symbolic (e.g., a poem, a feather) or concrete (e.g., a book, a potted plant). They can be modest—homemade cookies or bread, a music CD, flowers, or homegrown fruits—or more extravagant items such as opera or baseball season tickets or even truly excessive items like a piano, a car, or a large sum of money. Gifts can be appropriate or inappropriate in their type, monetary value, timing, content, frequency, intent of the giver, perception of the receiver, and their effect on the giver, receiver, or anyone else who may be affected by the gift-giving. Smolar (2003) broadened the concept of gift-giving in therapy and described several additional categories of therapists' gifts to clients: the gift of a transitional object, for example, a small rock or a shell or any token that clients can carry in a pocket or purse affirming the connection with the therapist between sessions; the gift of self-disclosure; the gift of (extra) time; the gift of physical touch; and the gift of presence.

Like self-disclosure and touch, the act of gift-giving is the act of crossing the traditionally drawn professional–interpersonal line. Clinically appropriate gift-giving by clients, therapists, or a third party is considered a boundary crossing. Appropriate gifts that are suitable expressions of clients' gratitude or given by therapists to clients as transitional objects to encourage or enhance the therapeutic alliance and that are of clinical benefit are also boundary crossings (Gutheil & Gabbard, 1993; Herlihy & Corey, 2006; Lazarus & Zur, 2002; Williams, 1997). Inappropriate gifts by clients, therapists, or third parties and gifts with inappropriate or offensive violent, sexual, racist, sexist, or homophobic themes are boundary violations. Inappropriately expensive gifts or any other gifts that create indebtedness, whether of therapist or client, are also boundary violations. Even small gifts can be inappropriate if, for example, they include inappropriate violent or sexual themes (Koocher & Keith-Spiegel, 1998). Gifts that create a conflict of interest, that are exploitative, or that negatively affect therapists' clinical effectiveness or clients' ability to benefit from treatment are boundary violations (Gutheil & Gabbard, 1998; Koocher & Keith-Spiegel, 1998; Zur, 2004b).

Each gift, whether from client or therapist, must be understood and evaluated within the context that it is given. Clients' personality, culture, economic status, and history determine the likely meaning of their gifts. The setting of therapy is also likely to shed light on the meaning and appropriateness of the gifts. The nature and quality of the therapeutic alliance are highly relevant, too, as gifts are primarily an expression of gratitude. As always, the timing and the main therapeutic orientation used would also determine the appropriateness of the gifts by clients or therapists. Culture-focused therapists, like humanistic and feminist-oriented psychotherapists, are more likely to give their clients gifts. Finally, the therapists' own culture and background are likely to have a bearing on the exchange of gifts in psychotherapy.

The Meaning of Clients' Gifts

Most psychotherapists do not view clients' gifts of small value, such as home-baked cookies or bread, books, CDs, or a potted plant, as clinically or ethically problematic (Borys, 1992; Borys & Pope, 1989; DeJulio & Berkman, 2003; Gerson & Fox, 1999; Pope, Keith-Spiegel, & Tabachnick, 1986; Shapiro & Ginzberg, 2003; Tabachnick, Keith-Spiegel, & Pope, 1991). Other appropriate gifts by clients include gifts to therapists after they have overcome a personal, medical, or other challenge such as pregnancy, an operation, or death of a family member. Pope, Tabachnick, and Keith-Spiegel (1987) labeled clients' gifts under $5 as "Behaviors that are almost universal" (p. 998). Generally, the gracious acceptance of small and symbolic gifts from clients has been viewed as enhancing the therapeutic alliance and is tied to positive clinical outcomes (Hahn, 1998; Herlihy & Corey, 2006; Spandler, Burman, Goldberg, Margison, & Amos, 2000; Zur, 2004a).

In contrast, expensive gifts, excessive gift-giving, insider stock market tips, or gifts given in the form of financial loans by clients have rung alarm bells for many therapists, ethicists, and licensing boards because these kinds of large gifts can easily affect therapists' objectivity and clinical effectiveness or create indebtedness (Herlihy & Corey, 2006; Lazarus & Zur, 2002; Williams, 1997). When such investment tips include inside information about a certain company stock, the matter becomes even more complicated because it may actually be illegal and unethical. One of the concerns with these kinds of gifts is the fact that the monetary value of such gifts cannot be calculated or known. National surveys of psychologists and social workers revealed that most therapists view the acceptance of gifts worth more than $50 from a client as ethically problematic (DeJulio & Berkman, 2003; Pope et al., 1987). As will be discussed later in this chapter, gifts that are made through bequests can also be fraught with obstacles and must be handled with care.

The meaning and appropriateness of clients' gifts have been central to the discussion of gifts. Most common, small, well-timed gifts have simply been viewed as a normal and healthy expression of gratitude. However, other gifts by clients have been fueled by motivations other than, or in addition to, gratitude. These may include attempts to express negative feelings, manipulate, or sexually seduce the therapists and similar behaviors. An important concern regarding gifts is whether a client's gift-giving is an effort to "buy" love. Many clients seek therapy because they do not feel appreciated, loved, or cared for. Others feel generally undeserving and have low self-esteem. One way that people who feel unworthy and not lovable can try to increase the chance of people, including therapists, liking them is through gift-giving. These clients often repeat such patterns with their lovers, friends, teachers, supervisors, employers, and other significant people in their lives (Knox, Hess, Williams, & Hill, 2003; Spandler et al., 2000).

Another motivation for gift-giving may be an attempt to have the therapist ally with a certain client rather than another. This is likely to be more common in couple, family, or group therapy and even more likely to occur in cases of child custody disputes.

Besides gifts given during the holidays and at termination, accepting a book, audiotape, CD, card, or poem that has special meaning to a client is common and usually acceptable. A baker may bring a loaf of bread to each session, and a farmer may do the same with some produce. A vet may offer a rescued puppy to a therapist who loves dogs, and a winemaker may give a case of his or her own prime wine to a therapist during the holidays. Similarly, artist clients often share their appreciation through gifts of their art. This may include a painting, sculpture, woven blanket, or handmade candle. Overinterpretation or needless discussion of the meaning of such naturally flowing gifts can be harming or insulting.

Gifts by clients can also be a way to try to deny, negate, or mask the client's negative feelings and maintain the continuity of a positive connection with the therapist. This kind of gift is likely to be given by a client to the therapist after the client missed a session or after a session when the two disagreed or argued on a certain topic or when the client feels slighted by the therapist (Hahn, 1998; Knox et al., 2003; Kritzberg, 1980; Spandler et al., 2000). It might also be given just before or right after a client abruptly terminates therapy against the therapist's advice. Obviously, gift-giving by clients can also be a way of acting out hostility, ambivalence, jealousy, competitiveness, and so on. As discussed later in the section on timing, paying attention to the timing of clients' gifts and, if necessary, discussing the subject with them is important.

Besides the clinical–psychological aspects, gift-giving in psychotherapy must always be viewed through the lens of the client's cultural background. Whereas in many Western cultures the verbal expression of gratitude seems appropriate and sufficient, in many non-Western cultures actual gifts and attendant rituals are the primary means of expressing gratitude, affirmation, and an emotional bond. Because, for the most part, gift-giving behavior derives from specific cultures, more often than not its meaning can only be understood within this cultural context (Corey, Corey, & Callahan, 2003; Koocher & Keith-Spiegel, 1998; Saad & Gill, 2003; Trimble, 2002). In Indian, Cambodian, and many other Asian cultures, there is greater focus on the meaning and rituals of gift-giving. In some of these cultures, the gift is not given to the person but to the spirit in the person. In others of that region, the gifts are perceived to be able to cure ailments or mental illness if the gifts appease the spirit of the ancestors carried by the sick person; according to this tradition, if the gift is not given, the sickness may return. In addition, gift-giving is a common practice in many Asian communities to show gratitude, respect, and the sealing of a relationship (Herlihy & Corey, 2006). Indian and many other cultures have very specific rituals regarding what should be given, when, to whom, and how. American Indian clients may give their therapist tobacco when asking for healing or, consistent with the rituals of giving gifts to healers, may give some other kind of gift at the very first session (American Indian Mental Health Advisory Council, 2004). Similarly, Jewish clients have been known to give Jewish cookbooks as a way to share their traditional cuisine with their therapists.

How Setting Affects the Meaning of Gifts

A gift from a client on an Indian reservation is most likely to have a different meaning from a gift given by a client in an urban setting. Some clinics and institutions choose to include a "no-gifts policy" in their office policies. As discussed subsequently, these policies may have an effect on the therapeutic process.

Regardless of the therapist's clinical or ethical stance on the subject of gifts, she or he must be aware that turning down a small gift may mean rejection or disrespect to an individual who comes from a culture that stresses hospitality, reciprocity, or the importance of gift-giving rituals. As was noted previously, a standard, preexisting no-gift policy is often meaningless and does not mitigate the sense of insult or humiliation for a non-Western client whose culture emphasizes the significance of gift-giving. The wise therapist will learn about each client's culture and gift-giving traditions, if possible, from the clients themselves.

Another complex issue is that of expensive gifts from wealthy clients. Therapists must take into consideration that wealthy clients are most often aware, consciously or unconsciously, of the significant impact of their wealth on other people and usually know from firsthand experience how power, influence, and social desirability go hand-in-hand with wealth. Gift-giving often has different meanings for the wealthy than for less prosperous individuals because frequently people have certain expectations, hopes, or fantasies regarding what affluent people can do for them (Gabbard & Nadelson, 1995). Expensive gifts, regardless of how financially insignificant they are for wealthy clients, can be a way to express gratitude but also a way to manipulate and control (Gabbard & Nadelson, 1995). Furthermore, costly gifts can be an unspoken quid pro quo, whereas others can represent a power play (Gabbard & Nadelson, 1995; Spandler et al., 2000). They can easily create indebtedness on the part of the therapist, which in turn is likely to impair the therapist's objectivity, confer a sense of obligation, and distort clinical judgment. As a result, such clients and therapists are in a difficult bind when it comes to gifts.

A therapist who is offered very expensive gifts by a wealthy client should not accept them regardless of how prosperous the client is. The fact that very expensive gifts are not a financial burden for wealthy clients is immaterial to the ethical aspect of accepting such presents. Instead of accepting these often tempting gifts, therapists must find ways to discuss their professional concerns with these clients and explain that such gifts make them uncomfortable. Nor should therapists be tempted to uncritically accept expensive gifts, such as theatre or baseball season tickets or a weekend at a client's vacation home, without discussing the meaning of the gift with the client and seeking consultation regarding its potential interference in the therapeutic process. If clients insist on giving very expensive gifts, therapists, with the help of consultation, may find creative arrangements with clients, such as making an anonymous donation to a mutually agreed-on charity. Awareness and, when appropriate, discussion of these concerns is of great importance and may be the only way to untangle often complicated webs. The meaning and impact of money vis-à-vis wealthy people is often an important clinical issue that can be brought to the surface, where it may generate discussion of the meaning of money in general, the clients' wealth in particular, and, when appropriate, their gift-giving. Although many well-to-do people may deny the importance of money and its effect on their lives, gift-giving can provide a precious opening for investigating such issues. Discussing with a wealthy client the meaning of a gift given by him or her can be well worth the effort in terms of shedding light on any issues the client may have associated with their social stature and influence.

Gifts by a Third Party and Medication Samples

Another type of gift in psychotherapy is that made by pharmaceutical companies as part of their multibillion dollar annual marketing efforts. Historically, it has been primarily psychiatrists who have been inundated by such gifts, but as psychologists have started gaining prescription privileges, the drug companies have increasingly targeted them, too. These gifts can be anything from pens and notepads, sample medications, free dinners, season tickets, all the way to free exotic golf vacations combined with free continuing education seminars. Psychiatry has demonstrated some of the pitfalls associated with the powerful influence and financial resources of pharmaceutical marketing. The literature on gift-giving by the pharmaceutical companies suggests that prescribing behavior is influenced by exposure to such marketing practices and identifies numerous ethical and professional concerns regarding conflicts of interest and practitioners' professional integrity (Polster, 2001; Reist & VandeCreek, 2004).

Medication samples include advertisements or promotional gifts by the pharmaceutical companies to medicating psychiatrists or psychologists who, in turn, commonly give them to their clients. This has been categorized by some as being a therapist's gift to a client (i.e., Gutheil & Gabbard, 1993). Giving medication samples can amount to a very "costly gift" if it involves expensive medication or is carried out over a long period of time. In fact, it can amount to thousands of dollars' worth of medication over a period of time. The concern with medication samples is twofold. The first concern is that the medicating therapist's relationship to the pharmaceutical companies and to the client, given the potential conflict of interest, is an ethically, and even clinically, problematic area (Polster, 2001; Reist & VandeCreek, 2004). The second concern is that, beside gratitude, clients may feel indebtedness toward the therapist who provides them with such medications gratis. It is hoped such concerns are addressed in therapy to reduce interference with the therapeutic process.

Gifts made in response to referrals of new clients, also called kickbacks, are unethical and often illegal (see chap. 5, this volume). The American Psychological Association (APA) Ethics Code states the following in Section 6.07:

> When psychologists pay, receive payment from, or divide fees with another professional, other than in an employer–employee relationship, the payment to each is based on the services provided (clinical, consultative, administrative, or other) and is not based on the referral itself. (2002, p. 1067, see also http://www.apa.org/ethics/code2002.html)

The concern with such gifts, especially if they are of significant monetary value or are made on an ongoing basis, is that they are part of an implicit business relationship, which creates indebtedness and conflicts of interest. Correspondingly, the issue has been addressed in federal and state laws, as well as in the bylaws and regulations of various organizations and corporations. Many solutions for these concerns seem to focus on limiting the value of the gifts (i.e., below $50) and on the requirement for disclosures.

Relatively common gifts from a third party involve gifts by a parent or a family member of a child–client. Such a gift is considered as a third-party gift if the giver is neither identified as a client nor involved in treatment. As with clients, appropriate gifts from a third party, such as baked goods for the holidays or at termination, are considered ethical and proper. Other third-party gifts may be given by someone related to a parent involved in a child custody or divorce dispute, or by someone who is associated with a client in individual, couple, family, or group therapy. This individual may want to positively influence the treating therapist in favor of the client or encourage the therapist to write a favorable evaluation or report on the client's behalf. Needless to say, such gifts from a third party should not be accepted.

Timing and Therapeutic Orientation

Timing of the gifts has also been considered an important factor in determining the meaning and appropriateness of gifts. As just mentioned, inexpensive gifts at holiday times and at termination have been deemed appropriate (Hahn, 1998; Herlihy & Corey, 2006; Shapiro & Ginzberg, 2003). A gift given by a client very early in therapy or after a difficult, confrontational, or missed session may require further discussion with the client. As was also noted earlier, expensive gifts given on the way to the door at the last session or after termination have also been reported as presenting therapists with ethical and clinical quandaries (Koocher & Keith-Spiegel, 1998).

Although analytically oriented therapists are likely to be concerned with the clinical effect of therapists' gift-giving on the analytic process, and especially countertransference considerations (Langs, 1982; Simon, 1991; Talan, 1989), there is wide agreement among most other therapists that following social conventions and giving appropriate small gifts for weddings or confirmations or giving gifts for clinical reasons is an acceptable practice (Corey et al., 2003; Fay, 2002; Gutheil & Gabbard, 1993). As in any clinical intervention, therapists are cautioned to be aware of their own motives when giving a gift and to be careful that the gifts are not attempts to get the client to like the therapist or to avoid conflict.

Therapists must also take into consideration that their clients, or those who are close to the clients, may misinterpret their gifts. Therapists' responses to clients' gifts are often tied closely to their theoretical orientation. The analytic schools often include avoidance of any boundary crossing that involves accepting or giving gifts to clients. The general, traditional analytic rule is that clients' gifts must be analyzed rather than received and that therapists who accept gifts are interfering in the transference analysis by acting out and gratifying an unconscious impulse (Bursten, 1959; Hahn, 1998; Kritzberg, 1980; Silber, 1969; Simon, 1991; Stein, 1965; Talan, 1989). In contrast, humanistic and feminist therapists have emphasized the importance of congruent relationships between therapists and clients, which are often enhanced by giving and receiving gifts (Greenspan, 1995; Jourard, 1971b; Williams, 1997, 2003). Behavioral, cognitive, cognitive–behavioral, family, and group therapies are likely to support appropriate gift-giving if they are likely to model healthy social exchange or enhance therapeutic effectiveness (Fay, 2002; Lazarus & Zur, 2002; Spandler et al., 2000). Gift-giving has also been viewed as a meaningful and clinically important part of the termination ritual in group therapy (Shapiro & Ginzberg, 2003).

When a therapist identifies a pattern or recognizes an important meaning, such as using gifts as a way to manipulate situations, to reduce tension that arises from disagreements, or to cover up hostile feelings, it is important, regardless of the theoretical orientation, to address these patterns with the client. When such a pattern manifests itself in the context of gift-giving, it may provide an opportunity to clinically work through and resolve these issues. Once the pattern is identified, there are many ways to incorporate it into the clinical work. These will be determined by the client, situation, timing, and the therapist's clinical orientation. If the therapist elects to bring it to the client's attention, it may be done in a constructive manner, which will cause neither embarrassment nor any sense of rejection (Knox et al., 2003; Spandler et al., 2000).

Therapists' Gifts

Therapists' gifts to clients have been given less attention than clients' gifts to therapists. Therapists' gifts, like clients' gifts, vary widely and may include a symbolic gift, such as a greeting card, or something more concrete, such as a book or CD (Corey et al., 2003; Reamer, 2001; Welfel, 2002). Many therapists' gifts are adjuncts to therapy as they either serve to enhance therapeutic alliance or are psychoeducational and complement the clinical work done in the office such as books, audiotapes, or CDs on mood swings for clients with bipolar disorder, meditation tapes for anxious clients, or educational brochures on stepfamilies for newlywed couples. Therapists often give gifts that serve as transitional objects, or they may give gifts that serve as clinical aids such as handwritten notes from the therapist with specific phrases or mantras to help clients dealing with anxiety, anger, despair, guilt, or dissociative states. The therapist may choose to follow social convention by giving gifts of affirmation or acknowledgment such as small graduation or wedding gifts; flowers or a card to a hospitalized client; a card for a grieving client; a supportive, reassuring gift (e.g., giving a flashlight to a child–client who is going on his first overnight camping trip); or a gift affirming the relationship (e.g., a souvenir from a trip abroad). Some other types of therapists' gifts that have been reported are offering a quarter for a parking meter, sharing a lunch with a client, or giving a client a ride to a nearby bus stop on a rainy day (Fay, 2002; Koocher & Keith-Spiegel, 1998; Lazarus, 1994).

Historically speaking, the question of therapists' gifts has been minimally explored since Freud struggled with it early in his career. When Freud realized that one of his clients was planning to buy a set of his complete works, he gave it to the client as a gift. Immediately following the gift-giving, Freud noticed that the patient's dreams seemed to be "drying up," and ever since then traditional analysis has held to the belief that gifts interfere with the natural course of analysis (Blanton, 1971).

Ethics and Keeping Records of Gift-Giving

Most professional organizations' codes of ethics do not address the issue of gifts directly. As was noted previously, the 2002 APA Ethics Code has an injunction against gifts for referrals, and the American Association for Marriage and Family Therapists (2001) Code of Ethics states, "Marriage and family therapists do not give to or receive from clients (a) gifts of substantial value or (b) gifts that impair the integrity or efficacy of the therapeutic relationship" (Section III, para. 10). Like any other ethical decision regarding boundary crossing, the decision whether to accept or give gifts should be based first and foremost on the welfare of the client and must be made under the general moral and ethical principles of beneficence and nonmaleficence. Applying these principles to gift-giving means that the decision should be clinically driven and must take into consideration clients' presenting problem, culture, history, age, and any other relevant client factors. As with any boundary crossing, when making the decision to accept or give a gift, the therapist should balance the risks against the benefits of accepting and not accepting a gift and, similarly, conduct a risk–benefit analysis for giving and not giving clients gifts. From a risk management point of view, gift exchanges such as self-disclosure, home visits, and nonsexual touch, have been cited as an area of concern (Gutheil & Gabbard, 1993; Williams, 1997). As with any risk management concern, therapists should consider documentation of any gifts as a way to protect themselves from misinterpretation of conduct.

Clients' or therapists' gifts should be documented in the clinical records. Modest gifts can be simply recorded as "Client presented me with small, handmade card featuring a soaring bird, symbolizing her newly found freedom." Or it could be more detailed, as in the following example:

> Upon termination and on the way to door of the last session, the (wealthy) client left an envelope with a $1,000 check in it. Consulting with Dr. X, an expert ethicist, confirmed my concern that it will be unethical and counterclinical for me to accept the gift. The check was sent back with a note thanking the client for the generous gift, explaining that my policies and professional guidelines prevent me from accepting it and proposing that if the client so wished, he could donate it to the charity of his choice. Client was told that I am open to discuss it further with him in person or on the phone.

Therapists' Responses to Clients' Gifts

The issue of whether therapists ought to discuss, question, interpret, or accept clients' gifts has been discussed extensively in the scholarly literature on gifts in psychotherapy. Therapists' responses obviously vary according to the type, timing, content, financial value, and appropriateness of the gift. As noted earlier, they also vary with therapists' therapeutic orientation and the meaning that they attach to clients' gift-giving.

A simple expression of gratitude, such as "Thank you," seems to be the most clinically and socially proper response to appropriate gifts. Although traditional analysis has discouraged therapists from accepting gifts, most clinicians and ethicists also agree that rejecting appropriate gifts of small monetary value but of highly symbolic and relational value can be offensive to clients, cause clients to feel rejected, and thus can be detrimental to the therapeutic alliance and the therapeutic process (Knox et al., 2003; Spandler et al., 2000). Massoth, a member of the 2004 APA Ethics Committee, stated "psychologists may do more harm than good if they refuse a reasonable gift" (Bailey, 2004, p. 62).

Because of the complexity of the potential meaning of gifts in therapy, as well as risk management considerations and the general lack of guidelines and education on these matters, many therapists are hesitant or reluctant to accept gifts from clients. A therapist's hesitation, uneasiness, or refusal to accept appropriate gifts can be easily interpreted as rejection, an experience that many clients are already too familiar with. Refusing a gift without attempting to understand the client's subjective reason for giving the gift is, at the minimum, a lost clinical opportunity. Some therapists, clinics, and institutions choose to include a "no-gifts policy" in their office policies. Such procedures may be ethical and legal, but from a clinical point of view it does not resolve concern with the negative impact that rejecting a gift may have on a client and the therapeutic process (Corey et al., 2003; Welfel, 2002).

At times, therapists may choose to accept small gifts, even though they seem to be an effort to manipulate the therapist; yet acceptance is preferable to shaming or insulting the clients, thereby causing a sense of rejection or irreversible disruption of therapy. Nonetheless, although therapists may accept such gifts, they must find a way to deal with the maladaptive gift-giving behaviors therapeutically. One idea is neither to accept the inappropriate gift nor to immediately interpret or reject it but instead to "hold" it for the time being. Hahn (1998) suggested that therapists in such situations may say, "I will keep the gift for now, but I'm not going to do anything with it until we have a chance to understand what it might be about" (p. 84). One hopes this approach will not result in any feeling of rejection in the client and at the same time does not miss the opportunity to explore the clinical concerns regarding the client's gift-giving patterns.

If a client expresses a wish to include the therapist in her or his will or trust, as a first step the therapist should reiterate that the clinical fee is all the compensation expected. Then, discussions should take place in which the meaning of this gift to the client is clarified and articulated. One solution for a client who insists on including his or her therapist in a will or trust is to have the client bequeath the money to a charity that is supported by both client and therapist.

When a therapist realizes after the fact that she or he was bequeathed money or assets by a client who died, it is necessary to seek consultation and navigate with caution around the concerns of confidentiality. A legal concern is that once the client is dead, it is too easy for relatives to claim undue influence. At that point, the therapist may, unfortunately, need to respond to civil malpractice lawsuits or to licensing board complaints initiated by the heirs. Without the client to set the record straight, the therapist is in an extremely vulnerable position. In a case in which the therapist's identity was not known to the relatives, confidentiality issues become highly relevant, which complicates the matter further and increases the therapist's vulnerability significantly. Another option for a therapist who is surprised by the gift is, if appropriate, to consider relinquishing or refusing the gift or proposing the anonymous donation option.

When receiving a gift from a client, a therapist must also take into consideration its potential effect on other people in the client's life. A precious family heirloom may have a sentimental value for a client's family members, and accepting such a gift may cause stress and ill feeling toward the client and the therapist.

Case Study: A Blessing in Disguise

A wealthy client presented her therapist with a very expensive leather jacket after the third month of therapy. After giving his courteous thanks for her expression of gratitude, the therapist invited her to share how she had decided to give that gift and what it meant to her. The ensuing discussion revealed a long history of the client's complex and tumultuous relationships to money. Being born into a wealthy family, she never trusted anyone for liking her for herself rather than for her money. From a very young age, she had learned how to "own" people by paying them or giving them expensive presents. She felt she had to buy love and care the same way her parents did. However, she insisted that the present to the therapist was different. The therapist was aware that he was in a bind. A basic risk–benefit analysis revealed that, on the one hand, rejecting the expensive gift for clinical and ethical reasons would be counterclinical as the client would be likely to feel rejected, ashamed, and even exposed and possibly quit therapy rather than face these feelings. On the other hand, accepting the gift could be equally counterclinical as it might very well reinforce her maladaptive patterns, reduce her trust in his true care for her, and as a result interfere with the therapeutic process. Pausing to consider and realizing the predicament he was in, the therapist decided to respond to the gift by first thanking her again and then proceeded to share with her frankly the difficult position in which he found himself. He expressed his ambiguous feelings, conflicting available options, and how he felt at a loss about what to do. The client was initially very upset and, in a fury of rejection, was ready to quit therapy. The therapist stayed calm and, in a compassionate way, told her that he understood how disappoint and insult it must be for her when he did not unquestioningly accept the gift. He articulated again his internal conflict about the gift. By that time, the client was a bit calmer and, in fact, was touched by the therapist's honestly expressed confusion about how to proceed, which mirrored her own internal struggles. Then, toward the end of the session, the therapist announced that he would "hold" the expensive gift until they had a chance to discuss it further. Over the next couple of sessions, the jacket was physically placed next to the therapist's and client's chairs and a fruitful discussion continued about the client's history, values, and attitudes toward money and how it affected her life. The client was still insisting, at that point, that the therapist should accept the gift. After a couple of months of further discussion of how money affected her relationships with people and fostered lack of trust in them, the client came to the realization that the jacket represented her "old" self. On her own, she decided to withdraw the gift.

12

Personal Space, Language, Silence, Clothing, Food, Lending, and Other Boundary Considerations

Thus far, in Part III, I have discussed self-disclosure, touch, and gifts as boundaries that exist within the therapeutic encounter, but many other types of interpersonal boundaries fall under the categories of verbal and nonverbal communication. These include space between therapists and clients, spoken language as well as the social "languages" of silence, clothing, food, lending and borrowing, and the exchange of cards. The boundary considerations of these issues are discussed in this chapter.

Space Between Therapists and Clients

The seating, or other spatial arrangement, represents a boundary between therapists and clients. Some therapists establish a clear physical boundary between themselves and their clients by sitting behind a desk while interviewing or consulting with clients. Others may establish the boundary between themselves and their clients by placement of a low coffee table. Many other therapists leave the space open and do not partition themselves from their clients with furniture. In contrast, traditional psychoanalysts sit out of sight behind the client who is lying on the analytic couch, establishing a visual boundary rather than a physical one. In special circumstances, such as prison settings, a therapist and a client may have a glass wall between them. Group therapists are likely to sit in a circle side by side with or opposite their clients, and psychoeducational-focused therapists may sit side by side with their client watching a video. Adventure or outdoor therapies, which involve backpacking, rope courses, or flying trapezes, have a very different spatial arrangement than the traditional therapy office. As with any boundary in therapy, the physical setting and any spatial arrangements between therapists and clients are always organized with clients' well-being in mind and can be understood within the context of therapy (i.e., the clients, setting, therapy, and therapist factors).

Actual distance between therapists and clients is another obvious expression of the extent of the boundary between therapists and clients. Like any boundary in therapy, it must be understood within the context of therapy. The therapist–client distance may change from client to client; for example, child clients may require or seek less distance than adult clients. Winnicott was reported by his client, Margaret Little, to hold her hands clasped between his through many hours as she lay on the couch, apparently in a near psychotic state (Little, 1990). Clients' gender and sexual orientations may also influence the distance that therapists or clients choose to sit from each other. Therapists may establish more distance when working with clients with borderline personality disorder or who are paranoid, volatile, or hostile. When it comes to seating arrangements and space between therapists and clients, therapists are not always in full control of the situation. As with touch and language, clients may or may not comply with therapists' established parameters and they may cross or violate therapists' set boundaries. A client with borderline personality disorder may violate the therapist's boundaries by inappropriate attempts to touch or kiss him or her. A paranoid client may choose to sit farther than the standard distance. Aggressive, hostile, or violent clients may attempt to intimidate therapists by "getting in their face" or being physically aggressive.

Many of the factors with regard to space reflect the same factors relating to touch discussed in chapter 10 of this volume. The setting of therapy determines what is an appropriate distance or spatial boundary between therapists and clients. Psychiatric medication evaluations and some forensic evaluations may be conducted in a more formal setting with more distance than other forms of therapy. Therapeutic orientation is another factor that determines the distance between therapists and clients. Humanistic or feminist-oriented therapists are likely to sit closer to their clients to reflect their focus on authentic and intimate therapist–client relationships. The traditional analytic setting in which therapists sit behind and out of clients' sight is significantly different, from a boundary and proximity point of view, than that of body psychotherapists who may use actual therapeutic touch with clients. Adventure or outdoor therapies also create different distances between therapists and clients who may be supporting each other on a rope course or otherwise interacting closely in a variety of activities. Distance can also vary within a session or from session to session with the same client. Within sessions, therapists and clients may start and end the session with a handshake and then settle for more distance during the session. The therapist may choose to go over and hold the hands or shoulders of a sobbing, grieving client or perhaps approach a client who has just announced a special accomplishment, such as receiving a diploma, and give the client a congratulatory pat on the back or high five. The 1980 movie, *Ordinary People,* directed by Robert Redford, demonstrated well how varying distance during therapy can be clinically effective. The therapist, played by Judd Hirsch, wheeled his chair far away from the client when he wanted to give the adolescent client, played by Timothy Hutton, space. A few seconds later, he wheeled it close up and confronted the teenager by being "in his face." The nature and quality of the therapeutic relationship is another factor that is likely to affect therapist–client distance. A closer and more intimate relationship is likely to naturally encourage closer proximity. Some therapists sit farther from their clients than others, reflecting not only their personal therapeutic orientation but also their own cultural and personal sense of comfort with space and proximity.

Spoken Language

Therapy has been dubbed the "talking cure," and spoken language is the primary tool of psychotherapists. Language, obviously, can help connect and heal, but it also can be a barrier between therapists and clients. Language has been considered a boundary issue and is usually discussed with regard to formalities, tone of voice, choice of words, type of language, and the use of silence (Gabbard & Nadelson, 1995; Gutheil & Gabbard, 1993). Language is an obvious boundary when therapists and clients do not speak the same language with the same fluency, when the spoken language is a second language for either client or therapist, or when dealing with clients who are hearing impaired.

The culture, class, and age of therapists and clients often determine the use of first name versus last name. More formal therapists or clients, or those from more European cultures as well as those who are older, are more likely to use the last name as a respectful way to address a client. Consistent with their therapeutic modality and their stance on therapeutic boundaries, feminist or humanistic therapists are more likely to ask clients to address them by their first name and use clients' first names rather than last as a way to reduce the power differential. National surveys of psychotherapists and clients revealed that most clients address therapists by their first name (Pope, Tabachnick, & Keith-Spiegel, 1987; Ramsdell & Ramsdell, 1993).

Tone of voice is another potential language variable as it can vary between businesslike and personal and between appropriate and inappropriately hostile, violent, or seductive. Likewise, choice of words is of extreme importance as it can connect people. Freud expressed his fondness for his patient Ferenczi by addressing him as "dear son." Therapists' use of jargon can be educational or distancing. Much has been written on the general health benefits of humor (e.g., Cousins, 1985; Galloway & Cropley, 1999), and several authors have discussed its use in psychotherapy (Fray & Salamen, 1997; Lemma, 1999; MacHovec, 1991). Like any form of language, humor can increase comfort and decrease anxiety, but it also can be offensive if it includes distasteful themes. Vulgar, abusive, sexist, racist, or other inappropriate, offensive language is a clear boundary violation (Gutheil & Gabbard, 1993). Inappropriate reference to a client's body parts can be a boundary violation as well (Gabbard & Nadelson, 1995).

Obviously, when therapists and clients are not equally fluent in the same language, there is a language barrier or boundary that separates them. The use of an interpreter who speaks the language or one who can help interpret for deaf clients brings a third party to the therapeutic exchange and can be helpful, destructive, or invasive. When the language used in therapy is a second language for either therapist or client, the nature of the barrier would depend on the verbal proficiency and cultural awareness of both. Even when client and therapist are both fluent in the language they speak to each other, the same words may have different meanings for each of them if they come from different cultures or socioeconomic classes. Language used without sensitivity to the vocabulary level of the listener can also create a barrier. Spoken language is a barrier if either therapist or client is hearing impaired unless both are fluent in signing.

Silence

Silence in therapy can be respectful, providing clients with the space they need to be quiet, to contemplate, to get in touch with memories or feelings, or to gather their thoughts. However, silence, which can be initiated by therapists or clients, can also be a form of therapeutic boundary as it may create a space between therapist and client. Silence can show respect, disrespect, abandonment, or hostility. The meaning of silence varies with people's cultures, personalities, mental disorders, emotional state, and age. The modality used in therapy and the quality and type of the therapeutic relationship are also likely to affect the perceived quality of the silence.

Clothing

Clothing has several boundary implications. On the most general and basic level, it serves as a boundary between people and their environment. Clothing also represents a social boundary between people and may signify professional or social status. Clothing varies with therapists' and clients' culture, climate, age, and the region they live in. A downtown New York City therapist is likely to dress differently and more formally from a therapist in a small, agricultural town where jeans are the clothes of choice. Therapists' clothing may also vary according to their therapeutic modality. Traditional psychoanalysts, for example, have a commitment to reduce variability, which may mean that they are likely to use neutral, conservative, and consistent clothing for sessions. Feminist and humanistic psychotherapists have a commitment to breaking interpersonal boundaries, which is likely to manifest itself in the wearing of casual and unique clothing.

Concerns with clothing have been cited in relation to clients or therapists wearing inappropriate or sexually suggestive clothing. Whether worn by therapist or client, it is likely to be a boundary violation because it tends to sexualize the therapeutic relationship. Overly casual clothing that is not suitable to the setting or is culturally insensitive can also be viewed as inappropriate, although not necessarily a boundary violation. Among Hindus, orthodox Jews, Muslims, and others, offense may be given when women wear clothing that reveals more than the face, hands, and feet, although such clothing is perfectly acceptable in Western or Latino cultures or in tropical regions. Clothing includes jewelry and printed T-shirts. Swastika pendants or offensive slogans or sayings on T-shirts can also be boundary violations. Displays of expensive jewelry or clothing can be an affiliative or distancing experience depending on the socioeconomic status of the clients or their sociopolitical values. As with language or nonverbal cues, clothing that is acceptable and appropriate to one person may promote affiliation or, conversely, be unacceptable and even offensive to others, creating a barrier. Therapists should be aware and thoughtful about the message they give with the way they dress and also should discuss with clients when clients' dress seems offensive or inappropriate.

Sharing Food With Clients

Food is inherently a nourishing and nurturing experience. Sharing food is universally considered a communal or bonding experience, a gesture of bringing people together. It reduces interpersonal boundaries and enhances communal ones. The giving and receiving of food in psychotherapy includes clients' gifts of home-baked goods, sharing ethnic cuisine, and special foods given around the holiday season. Some therapists provide drinks and candy in the waiting room as a way of extending a warm reception. Others may offer it in the consulting room, which is a more specific, individual gesture or even clinical intervention. Sharing food with clients with eating disorders has been reported by a number of therapists from different orientations. In this case, the sharing of food is part of the treatment plan and is done exclusively and specifically for clinical treatment purposes. As mentioned earlier, there are family therapists who use the "anorexic lunch," whereby a therapist goes to a restaurant with an anorexic client to observe and intervene with the client's eating behavior (Fay, 2002; Minuchin, 1974). Therapists may offer a small cake or cupcake with candles to celebrate birthdays of clients who are isolated and who have neither family members nor friends to commemorate the event.

Our predecessors introduced us to the idea of therapists breaking bread with clients as a way to enhance therapeutic relationships and connect better with their clients. Freud fed the client known as the Rat Man (Isaac, 2004), and Winnicott ended some of his sessions with coffee and biscuits (Little, 1990). More recently, Lazarus (1994) and Fay (2002) discussed the positive clinical impact of sharing a lunch or dinner with clients. Surveyed psychologists reported that about 11% of them went to eat with clients after sessions (Borys & Pope, 1989); nevertheless, according to other authors, eating out with a client was generally viewed as unethical behavior (Baer & Murdock, 1995; Gutheil & Gabbard, 1993). A survey of clients revealed that about 10% of psychotherapists shared a meal with clients, 46% of the clients viewed the sharing as having no effect on therapy, 43% viewed it as somewhat or very detrimental, and 10% viewed it as somewhat or very beneficial (Ramsdell & Ramsdell, 1993). A more recent national survey of social workers (DeJulio & Berkman, 2003) revealed that 68% responded that going out to eat with a client was ethical under either some or rare conditions, and only 27% responded that it was never ethical. As with any other boundary crossing, therapists should conduct a risk–benefit analysis when deciding whether to eat out with a client; their ethical decision should take into consideration the context of therapy and the welfare of the client.

Sharing food, as was discussed in chapter 6 of this volume, is also a frequent occurrence when therapists conduct home visits and the family offers them tea and cookies or a full dinner. Refusing an offer to share food with the family during a home visit is likely to be perceived as insulting or, at least, discourteous, and is very likely to negatively affect the therapeutic alliance, trust, and clinical efficacy. Similarly, sharing food is an unavoidable practice in adventure or outdoor therapy.

Lending and Borrowing

Lending items to another person is a form of nonverbal communication. Because it is usually expected that the item lent will be returned within a certain time frame, the act of lending communicates the expectation that there will be an ongoing relationship. Lending and borrowing in therapy can take place in either direction, between client and therapist or vice versa. Most often the items will be books, music CDs or audiotapes, poetry, art collection books, or film videos. Therapists often lend books, music, audiotapes, CDs, and videos to clients for educational enrichment and to provide emotional support. Lending a book on stepfamilies may be helpful to a newly wedded couple with children from former marriages. Lending a relaxation CD may help a client unwind. Lending a self-help book on depression or dealing with obsession can be effective in educating clients on using cognitive–behavioral techniques for dealing with their problems. Many clients lend music CDs, poetry, or art books to their therapists to help the therapists understand them better. These items often have a deep, emotional meaning for clients, which compel clients to share them with their therapists.

Freud not only gave gifts to his clients but also lent them books (Gutheil & Gabbard, 1993). More recently, Lazarus (1994) and Fay (2002) have discussed the positive impact that lending has on the therapeutic alliance and progress in therapy. Lending by either therapists or clients is a boundary crossing because it involves an exchange of items that are not money (which is the standard expectation) and goes beyond the standard or customary therapeutic therapist–client boundary. A second type of boundary involved in such transactions is the boundary established by the inherent understanding that the lent object must be returned to the lender.

As with any boundary crossing or clinical intervention, therapists must have a clear clinical rationale when lending an object to a client. Such lending must be made with full consideration of all the client's relevant personal factors. As with gifts, clinicians must pay attention to the meaning and intent of the lending and its implications for the therapeutic process. For example, when a therapist lends items from her professional resources, such as a book on autism to a client whose child is autistic and who is receiving therapy to help the client cope with the child's care needs, what has been communicated is fairly clear, whether or not it is stated aloud: "I think this might help you, and we can use it as material for discussion in your ongoing course of therapy." However, when a therapist loans a client something from his or her personal stores, such as a CD of relaxing music, unless the clinical rationale is made clear, the client (depending on cultural factors and presenting problem) might perceive that the therapist is initiating a more personal level of relationship outside the therapeutic one.

Boundaries can also be crossed when the lending agreement is not upheld, when therapists or clients do not return the items on time or not at all. To avoid these kinds of violations and the clinical fallout that is likely to follow, therapists must communicate and clarify the lending terms before or as it takes place. Ambiguous arrangements are likely to lead to ambiguous boundaries, misunderstandings, disappointments, and a potentially negative impact on the therapeutic alliance and clinical efficacy.

Greeting and Sympathy Cards

Sending or giving a greeting or sympathy card is geared to mark life transitions such as a graduation, wedding, birth, holiday, birthday, confirmation, bar mitzvah, death, illness, hospitalization, or recovery. It can also mark the termination of therapy or celebrate the client overcoming a challenge with the aid of therapy. Such cards are most often sent or given by therapists and clients but can also be sent by parents of a child who is in therapy or by a third party, such as a pharmacology company. Child clients often draw or color pictures as cards for their therapists. Exchanging greeting or sympathy cards is a boundary issue, because it goes beyond the standard therapeutic exchange.

As with sharing meals, lending books, and gift-giving, Freud also was reported to have sent his patients postcards (Gutheil & Gabbard, 1993). Of psychologists surveyed, about 20% reported sending greeting cards to their clients (D. H. Lamb & Catanzaro, 1998). When therapists send greeting or sympathy cards to clients, they must treat it like any clinical intervention or gift-giving and, of course, take into account all those important client factors again. Unless the cards are related to events that are part of therapy, a client's greeting or sympathy cards are likely to correspond to the therapist's level of self-disclosure. Unless therapists reveal a birthday, marriage, illness, birth of a child, or other personal information to their clients, the clients are not likely to have enough information to send cards to their therapists. Accepting cards from clients is very similar to accepting gifts, whereby the meaning, propriety, and intent should be examined. Although most greeting and sympathy cards are likely to be appropriate, therapists should note when improper sexual, violent, sexist, racist, or any offensive themes are included in the card and respond suitably. As with gift-giving, the correctness and the meaning of the cards are likely to be related to the therapist's or the client's culture, personality, gender, and age. Appropriate cards by either therapists or clients are boundary crossings and, as such, can enhance the therapeutic alliance and clinical efficacy. Inappropriate or offensive cards are boundary violations.

Case Study: From Cupcake to Sculpture—
Many Ways to Communicate

A male therapist has been working with an executive who is a socially isolated, dysthymic female client who is nevertheless fully oriented to reality and has a general tendency to intellectualize, stay superficial, and avoid deep and authentic feelings. The therapist noticed that every time the client faced emotionally charged issues she started analyzing them and became emotionally flat.

At times, it sounded like she was talking about someone else rather than about herself. The therapist's office was organized in such a way that there was no furniture between the client's chair and the therapist's chair, and his chair was easily movable. After a couple of months of therapy, in response to the client intellectualizing a major emotional event in her life, the therapist stated, "I want to encourage you to stay with yourself or go within yourself and experience your feelings quietly. I'm going to move in closer, if it is okay with you, to help you remember that I'm with you as you do that." The idea is that the closer proximity may create a sense of connection that is not based on cognition or spoken words; it also may promote an emotionally safe environment that may enable the client to get in touch with and stay with her feelings. He moved closer after he received a nod of approval. Prior to that intervention, the therapist had to make a careful risk–benefit analysis. Against the benefit of helping the client tolerate the silence and get in touch with her feelings, the therapist weighed the concern that, given the gender differences, proposing a silent moment and a closer proximity to the client might be seen as suggestive. He took care to get her permission to come closer before he did. The intervention seemed successful as the client appeared to be surprised and appreciative of his attentiveness to her physical and acoustic boundaries. The client gradually learned to articulate and stay with her feelings more successfully.

A few months later, the client's birthday was approaching. The therapist was aware that the client was isolated and had neither close friends nor family in the area. He was contemplating whether to acknowledge her birthday by giving her a simple birthday card and a cake with candles. His concern was that such a gesture may be perceived as a crossover from the clinical to the social and may bring about a feeling of indebtedness on behalf of the client. However, having the client deal with an emotional rather than an intellectual experience was perfectly in line with their clinical work. In addition, the clinic, at which he was on staff, had a no-gift policy. He consulted with the clinic director, who gave him permission and suggested that he give the client a birthday card and present her with a cupcake and a candle rather than a cake, which seemed to be too extravagant. The consultation and risk–benefit analysis resulted in his presenting his surprise celebration by stating, "I don't often do this because most people have friends and family but you have no one near right now and you are certainly worthy of celebration."

Sometime later in therapy, the therapist was about to go on a scheduled vacation. At that time, the client had already developed some dependency on the therapist and her feelings of abandonment were triggered by the upcoming separation. Again in consultation with the clinic director, he decided to lend her a tiny, wooden sculpture from his office that she had always admired to serve as a transitional object so she could feel some connection to the therapist while he was away from the office. Prior to offering the client the sculpture, the therapist had to weigh the benefit of providing her with a transitional object to help her deal with the separation and engage her in an emotional experience against the risk that the sculpture might break or get lost and the client's potential negative feelings if either event should happen. He also considered the remote possibility that the sculpture might not be returned. Ultimately, the client endured the separation more comfortably, and the sculpture was returned intact.

IV

Final Thoughts

13

Toward a Better Understanding of Boundaries in Therapy

This book confronts one of the most complex, controversial, and puzzling issues in psychotherapy, the subject of psychotherapeutic boundaries. Since Freud's time, practitioners have been debating whether therapists should touch their clients, accept their gifts, self-disclose to them, or socialize with them. Beyond the agreement that therapists should never be sexual with their clients, should attempt to "do no harm," honor their clients' privacy, and treat them with dignity and respect, there is very little agreement on what constitutes appropriate behavior when it comes to boundaries. In fact, there is no agreement on the meaning of therapeutic boundaries, what constitutes appropriate psychotherapeutic boundaries, and what their proper clinical and ethical applications are.

Boundaries are extremely important in psychotherapy because they define the fiduciary relationships and the therapeutic frame. Boundaries that deal with issues of time, money, and place define the boundary around the therapeutic relationships and differentiate it from social or other relationships. Boundaries that define and determine the type and quality of therapist–client interactions include physical contact and proximity, therapists' self-disclosure, exchange of gifts, bartering, and different types of dual relationships. Although maintaining appropriate boundaries is the prime responsibility of therapists, clients also contribute to and define the nature and development of therapeutic boundaries.

Therapists must realize that many boundary crossings are unavoidable, such as therapists' spoken or unspoken self-disclosure, and must take this fact into consideration. Intentional crossing of other boundaries can be of extreme importance for therapeutic efficacy. This includes appropriate supportive touch, gracious acceptance of appropriate gifts, making a home visit to a homebound client or a hospital visit to an ill client, and intentional self-disclosure for the purpose of modeling or enhancing authenticity. Rigid avoidance of such boundary crossing is likely to result in a low quality of therapeutic alliance, which is the best predictor of therapeutic outcome.

There are times, however, when therapists must avoid crossing boundaries if it could reasonably be expected to impair the psychologist's objectivity, competence, or effectiveness in performing his or her job or seems likely to harm the client or interfere with therapeutic effectiveness. These include prematurely touching a client with a long history of sexual trauma, making a home visit to an able client with borderline personality disorder who can benefit from clear and consistent boundaries rather than flexible ones, bartering with a narcissistic and entitled client, or accepting a very expensive or otherwise inappropriate gift.

Similarly, engaging in a dual relationship can be unavoidable and common, helpful, benign, or damaging. Dual relationships in rural, military, forensic, and many such small communities are unavoidable and should be taken into account clinically. Dual relationships are a common and normal part of small ethnic and other minority or spiritual communities. Therapists must carefully weigh the risks and benefits of engaging in such relationships as they can become complex and hard to manage. Any dual relationship that could reasonably be expected to impair the psychologist's objectivity and competence, be exploitative to the client, create a conflict-of-interest situation, or interfere with the therapist's clinical duties, should be avoided. Needless to say, sexual dual relationships with clients are always unethical and often illegal.

The aim of this book is to help therapists make informed decisions with regard to the ethical application of clinically appropriate therapeutic boundaries. To achieve this goal, the book provides the information and background regarding each type of boundary crossing and provides a decision-making process to guide therapists. The application of boundaries in therapy should be based on the context of therapy. That means that whether to self-disclose, touch clients, conduct therapy via e-mail, barter, and so on all depends on four factors:

- ☐ the client's presenting problem, culture, age, gender, and history;
- ☐ the setting where therapy takes place, which includes location, type of setting or institution, and the culture;
- ☐ therapy, which involves the therapeutic orientation used; length, type, frequency, and intensity of therapy; and the quality of the therapeutic relationships; and
- ☐ therapists' factors, such as age, gender, culture, and training or scope of practice.

A carefully documented decision-making process, with complete clinical records, treatment plan, and record of all consultations, will answer any clinical and risk management concerns regarding boundary crossing without compromising clinical integrity. The decision-making process regarding boundaries in therapy should rely on critical thinking principles, risk–benefit analysis, concerns with clients' autonomy, the principle of "do no harm," and the therapist's responsibility to contribute to the welfare of the client with justice and fidelity.

By tailoring boundary crossings to the unique, specific situation of each client and context of therapy, therapists may feel an abiding satisfaction in the knowledge that every decision was meticulously formed to assure the best possible care for those we have sworn to serve and whose lives it is our mission to lift up.

Appendix A

Examples of Boundary Crossings and Boundary Violations in Psychotherapy

This appendix provides examples of certain situations that may constitute boundary crossings or boundary violations by therapists. The table is intended as an extension of prior reading or discussion and can be used as a teaching tool or as a guide for reflection and professional dialogue. Consider each situation, keeping in mind the context factors—client, therapist, theoretical therapeutic relationship, and setting—that might be in play. Some questions for reflection and conversation include the following:

- [ ] Are there situations when the client may need to be informed that an action constitutes a boundary violation, given the context?
- [ ] If any of the examples of boundary violations seem blatant or obvious, can you think of context factors that might cloud this, in the mind of a therapist?
- [ ] When might a boundary be crossed or violated by inaction rather than action?
- [ ] Are there situations in which a boundary violation is likely, regardless of the therapist's good intent?
- [ ] What proactive steps can therapists take to avoid boundary violations or to broaden their limits of competence enough to step out on a limb if it will help the client?

Situation (alphabetical by topic)	Boundary crossing: Approach with care	Boundary violation: Avoid
Bartering: Client offers to barter housecleaning services in exchange for therapy services.	The client's insurance does not cover therapy and the regular fee is too high. Client is too proud to accept free therapy and the therapist and client agree on an hour-for-hour work exchange.	The therapist unnecessarily extends treatment to continue receiving housecleaning services.
Bartering: Client barters an antique lamp for therapy services.	The client is an antique collector and barters the lamp for fair market value as established by an appraiser. He offers a dollar-for-dollar, goods-for-service exchange.	The therapist learns that the lamp is a priceless family heirloom and the barter is likely to upset the client's family members but agrees to the exchange anyway.
Clothing: A woman therapist wears a short-sleeved blouse during a client session.	The client is uncomfortable seeking help from a professional and stranger, so the therapist chooses climate- and culture-appropriate, informal clothing to help break down the interpersonal barrier.	The therapist changes into a highly revealing blouse because she tries to look attractive to the client who she is about to have a session with.
Dual relationship: Therapist smokes peyote with client.	A therapist who practices on an Indian reservation accepts—after an extensive discussion of potential risks—a client's invitation to a traditional Navajo peyote ceremony.	A therapist joins a client to recreationally use peyote or other psychedelic substances.
Dual relationship: Therapist sees a therapist–colleague for therapy.	The therapist's and client's only other regular contact outside therapy is at large annual professional conferences.	The client is a very close colleague, a member of the therapist's peer supervision group, and they share a few clients.
Dual relationship: Therapist and former client are also lovers.	Ten years after terminating short-term therapy for work–life balance issues, a therapist and her	The therapist and client terminate therapy in order to engage in a sexual relationship.

	former high-functioning client meet by chance, begin a social relationship, engage in premarital counseling, and finally decide to marry.	
Dual relationship: Therapist and client are both members of the same congregation.	The therapist treats a fellow member of the congregation who she sees sometimes at Sunday mass.	The therapist treats a couple who plans to divorce and are engaged in a bitter custody dispute over their son. The therapist also leads a prayer group at the congregation where one client attends services.
Gifts: Client gives therapist an inexpensive, small gift.	A teenage client often clashes with his parents over his music choices, so the therapist agrees when the client asks to burn a CD of his favorite music for her in hopes that she will like the music.	The therapist enthusiastically accepts a CD with sexually offensive and violent lyrics from a client without a discussion or feedback.
Gifts: Therapist gives client a gift before leaving on vacation.	The therapist gives a client who experiences separation anxiety a symbolic gift of a small rock to help him deal with feelings of abandonment during the therapist's vacation.	The therapist gives a client a bouquet of flowers to help assuage guilt feelings for going on vacation.
Gifts: Parents of a client give a gift to the therapist.	Parents of a young child express their appreciation by sending home-baked cookies to the child's therapist.	A therapist who is helping a couple to deal with divorce and custody conflicts accepts an expensive gift of season tickets from one of the parents.
Home office: Therapist sees client in her home.	The therapist's entire practice is at her home. She sees clients there after thorough screenings and obtaining informed consents.	The therapist invites a certain client, to whom she is attracted, to her home rather than her standard office for a session.
Home visit: Therapist meets a client in client's home.	The therapist meets with an elderly, housebound, dying	The therapist meets a client, who professes her attraction to him, in

continued

Situation (alphabetical by topic)	Boundary crossing: approach with care	Boundary violation: Avoid
	client at the client's home.	her house when the client's husband is on a business trip.
Language: Therapist uses profanities.	The therapist uses profanity rarely and only when acknowledging a client's feelings, choosing to do so because it mirrors the client's own language that she uses to express feelings.	The therapist uses profanity to express frustration with a client who, in her opinion, is not putting forth any effort to progress along the mutually agreed on treatment plan.
Out-of-office encounter: Client and therapist see each other partially clothed.	The therapist and client unexpectedly see each other partially clothed in a locker room of a local gym. The therapist takes the cue from the client, gets dressed, and does not initiate a conversation.	The therapist invites a client to a hot-tub party where people are either nude or partially clothed.
Place for therapy: Therapist and client have a therapy session in a nearby park.	The therapist uses in vivo desensitization with an agoraphobic client.	The therapist takes a client, who previously professed her attraction to him, to an evening walk in a nearby park.
Self-disclosure: Therapist is upset with a client and says so to the client.	The therapist expresses controlled anger at a client who, in a fit of rage, broke the therapist's treasured sculpture. The therapist explains what the sculpture symbolizes to her, as a way of teaching the client to think before acting.	When a client discloses that she has cut herself again, the therapist turns red and sputters, "My own sister killed herself that way! Do you think I'm going to stand by and watch you do the same thing?"
Self-disclosure: Therapist discloses to a client that he also experienced depression.	The therapist minimally and appropriately discloses about his depression and how he overcame it as a way of modeling with a depressed client.	The therapist discloses extensively to a client about his depression to elicit sympathy and justify missing sessions without notice.
Time: Therapist provides a 3-hour session.	The therapist schedules a 3-hour session with a large family whose members have	The therapist schedules a 3-hour session with a wealthy client because the therapist is behind

	gathered from all over the country specifically for this event.	in his house payment and needs extra cash.
Time: A client requests a 9:30 p.m. start time for therapy sessions.	This time slot is the only one that will work given the client's other obligations, such as a long commute and having to pick up his child from child care.	The therapist agrees to the time slot requested even though the client stated it would be more romantic to meet late in the day when other office staff is not present. The therapist plans to use the session time to discuss attraction issues.
Touch: Therapist touches client forcefully.	The therapist physically stops a client from violently banging his head on the wall.	A female therapist shoves a male client in anger to teach him that not all women conform to his ideal of weakness.
Touch: Therapist embraces a client.	The therapist reciprocates a warm greeting embrace as a culturally sensitive response to a client.	The therapist reciprocates a seductive full-body embrace by a female client because he fears the client will terminate therapy if he "freezes up."
Touch: Therapist strokes the hair of a client.	The therapist visits a terminally ill client in the hospital and strokes the client's hair, at her request, while saying a final goodbye.	The therapist strokes a client's hair as a way of helping her come to terms with her sexual feelings.

Appendix

B

Ethics Codes on Boundaries and Dual Relationships in Psychotherapy and Counseling

This appendix provides direct quotes from, and references to, the major, national professional organizations' codes of ethics on the following boundary considerations: nonsexual dual relationships, bartering, gifts, and nonsexual touch. For each of these four topics, the following organizations' ethics codes are presented: American Psychological Association (2002), National Association of Social Workers (1999), American Psychiatric Association (2001), American Association of Marriage and Family Therapists (2001), and American Counseling Association (2005).

Dual or Multiple (Nonsexual) Relationships

American Psychological Association "Ethical Principles of Psychologists and Code of Conduct" (2002)
Section 3.05 Multiple Relationships

(a) A multiple relationship occurs when a psychologist is in a professional role with a person and (1) at the same time is in another role with the same person, (2) at the same time is in a relationship with a person closely associated with or related to the person with whom the psychologist has the professional relationship, or (3) promises to enter into another relationship in the future with the person or a person closely associated with or related to the person.

A psychologist refrains from entering into a multiple relationship if the multiple relationship could reasonably be expected to impair the psychologist's objectivity, competence, or effectiveness in performing his or her functions as a psychologist, or otherwise risks exploitation or harm to the person with whom the professional relationship exists.

Multiple relationships that would not reasonably be expected to cause impairment or risk exploitation or harm are not unethical.

(b) If a psychologist finds that, due to unforeseen factors, a potentially harmful multiple relationship has arisen, the psychologist takes reasonable steps to resolve it with due regard for the best interests of the affected person and maximal compliance with the Ethics Code.

(c) When psychologists are required by law, institutional policy, or extraordinary circumstances to serve in more than one role in judicial or administrative proceedings, at the outset they clarify role expectations and the extent of confidentiality and thereafter as changes occur. (See also Standards 3.04, Avoiding Harm, and 3.07, Third-Party Requests for Services.)

National Association of Social Workers *Code of Ethics* (1999)
1.06 Conflict of Interest

(c) Social workers should not engage in dual or multiple relationships with clients or former clients in which there is a risk of exploitation or potential harm to the client. In instances when dual or multiple relationships are unavoidable, social workers should take steps to protect clients and are responsible for setting clear, appropriate, and culturally sensitive boundaries. (Dual or multiple relationships occur when social workers relate to clients in more than one relationship, whether professional, social, or business. Dual or multiple relationships can occur simultaneously or consecutively.)

American Psychiatric Association *Principles of Medical Ethics With Annotations Especially Applicable to Psychiatry* (2001)
This code does not mention dual or multiple relationships.

American Association of Marriage and Family Therapists *Code of Ethics* (2001)
Principle I: Responsibility to Clients
1.3. Marriage and family therapists are aware of their influential positions with respect to clients, and they avoid exploiting the trust and dependency of such persons. Therapists, therefore, make every effort to avoid conditions and multiple relationships with clients that could impair professional judgment or increase the risk of exploitation. Such relationships include, but are not limited to, business or close personal relationships with a client or the client's immediate family. When the risk of impairment or exploitation exists due to conditions or multiple roles, therapists take appropriate precautions.

American Counseling Association *Code of Ethics* (2005)

A.5.c. Nonprofessional Interactions or Relationships (Other Than Sexual or Romantic Interactions or Relationships)
Counselor–client nonprofessional relationships with clients, former clients, their romantic partners, or their family members should be avoided, except when the interaction is potentially beneficial to the client. (See A.5.d.)

A.5.d. Potentially Beneficial Interactions
When a counselor–client nonprofessional interaction with a client or former client may be potentially beneficial to the client or former client, the counselor must document in case records, prior to the interaction (when feasible), the rationale for such an interaction, the potential benefit, and anticipated consequences for the client or former client and other individuals significantly involved with the client or former client. Such interactions should be initiated with appropriate client consent. Where unintentional harm occurs to the client or former client, or to an individual significantly involved with the client or former client, due to the nonprofessional interaction, the counselor must show evidence of an attempt to remedy such harm. Examples of potentially beneficial interactions include, but are not limited to, attending a formal ceremony (e.g., a wedding/commitment ceremony or graduation); purchasing a service or product provided by a client or former

client (excepting unrestricted bartering); hospital visits to an ill family member; mutual membership in a professional association, organization, or community. (See A.5.c)

A.5.e. Role Changes in the Professional Relationship

When a counselor changes a role from the original or most recent contracted relationship, he or she obtains informed consent from the client and explains the right of the client to refuse services related to the change. Examples of role changes include

1. changing from individual to relationship or family counseling, or vice versa;
2. changing from a nonforensic evaluative role to a therapeutic role, or vice versa;
3. changing from a counselor to a researcher role (i.e., enlisting clients as research participants), or vice versa; and
4. changing from a counselor to a mediator role, or vice versa.

Clients must be fully informed of any anticipated consequences (e.g., financial, legal, personal, or therapeutic) of counselor role changes.

A.6.a. Advocacy

When appropriate, counselors advocate at individual, group, institutional, and societal levels to examine potential barriers and obstacles that inhibit access and/or the growth and development of clients.

A.6.b. Confidentiality and Advocacy

Counselors obtain client consent prior to engaging in advocacy efforts on behalf of an identifiable client to improve the provision of services and to work toward removal of systemic barriers or obstacles that inhibit client access, growth, and development.

A.7. Multiple Clients

When a counselor agrees to provide counseling services to two or more persons who have a relationship, the counselor clarifies at the outset which person or persons are clients and the nature of the relationships the counselor will have with each involved person. If it becomes apparent that the counselor may be called upon to perform potentially conflicting roles, the counselor will clarify, adjust, or withdraw from roles appropriately. (See A.8.a., B.4.)

Bartering

American Psychological Association "Ethical Principles of Psychologists and Code of Conduct" (2002)
6.05 Barter With Clients/Patients
Barter is the acceptance of goods, services, or other nonmonetary remuneration from clients/patients in return for psychological services. Psychologists may barter only if (1) it is not clinically contraindicated, and (2) the resulting arrangement is not exploitative. (See also Standards 3.05, Multiple Relationships, and 6.04, Fees and Financial Arrangements.)

National Association of Social Workers *Code of Ethics* (1999)
1.13 Payment for Services
(a) When setting fees, social workers should ensure that the fees are fair, reasonable, and commensurate with the services performed. Consideration should be given to clients' ability to pay.
(b) Social workers should avoid accepting goods or services from clients as payment for professional services. Bartering arrangements, particularly involving services, create the potential for conflicts of interest, exploitation, and inappropriate boundaries in social workers' relationships with clients. Social workers should explore and may participate in bartering only in very limited circumstances when it can be demonstrated that such arrangements are an accepted practice among professionals in the local community, considered to be essential for the provision of services, negotiated without coercion, and entered into at the client's initiative and with the client's informed consent. Social workers who accept goods or services from clients as payment for professional services assume the full burden of demonstrating that this arrangement will not be detrimental to the client or the professional relationship.

American Psychiatric Association *Principles of Medical Ethics With Annotations Especially Applicable to Psychiatry* (2001)
This code does not mention bartering.

American Association of Marriage and Family Therapists *Code of Ethics* (2001)
Principle VII: Financial Arrangements
    7.5. Marriage and family therapists ordinarily refrain from accepting goods and services from clients in return for services rendered. Bartering for professional services may be conducted only if: (a) the supervisee or client requests it, (b) the relationship is not exploitative, (c) the professional relationship is not distorted, and (d) a clear written contract is established.

American Counseling Association *Code of Ethics* (2005)
A.10.d. Bartering
    Counselors may barter only if the relationship is not exploitive or harmful and does not place the counselor in an unfair advantage, if the client requests it, and if such arrangements are an accepted practice among professionals in the community. Counselors consider the cultural implications of bartering and discuss relevant concerns with clients and document such agreements in a clear written contract.

Gifts

American Psychological Association "Ethical Principles of Psychologists and Code of Conduct" (2002)
    This code does not mention gifts.

National Association of Social Workers *Code of Ethics* (1999)
    This code does not mention gifts.

American Psychiatric Association *Principles of Medical Ethics With Annotations Especially Applicable to Psychiatry* (2001)
    This code does not mention gifts.

American Association of Marriage and Family Therapists *Code of Ethics* (2001)
Principle III: Professional Competence and Integrity
    3.10. Marriage and family therapists do not give to or receive from clients (a) gifts of substantial value or (b) gifts that impair the integrity or efficacy of the therapeutic relationship.

American Counseling Association *Code of Ethics* (2005)
A.10.e. Receiving Gifts
  Counselors understand the challenges of accepting gifts from clients and recognize that in some cultures, small gifts are a token of respect and showing gratitude. When determining whether or not to accept a gift from clients, counselors take into account the therapeutic relationship, the monetary value of the gift, a client's motivation for giving the gift, and the counselor's motivation for wanting or declining the gift.

Nonsexual Touch

American Psychological Association "Ethical Principles of Psychologists and Code of Conduct" (2002)
  This code does not mention nonsexual touch.

National Association of Social Workers *Code of Ethics* (1999)
1.10 Physical Contact
  Social workers should not engage in physical contact with clients when there is a possibility of psychological harm to the client as a result of the contact (such as cradling or caressing clients). Social workers who engage in appropriate physical contact with clients are responsible for setting clear, appropriate, and culturally sensitive boundaries that govern such physical contact.

American Psychiatric Association *Principles of Medical Ethics With Annotations Especially Applicable to Psychiatry* (2001)
  This code does not mention nonsexual touch.

American Association of Marriage and Family Therapists *Code of Ethics* (2001)
  This code does not mention nonsexual touch.

American Counseling Association *Code of Ethics* (2005)
  This code does not mention nonsexual touch.

References

Adoption Assistance and Child Welfare Act of 1980, Pub. L. No. 96-272. 94, U.S.C. § 500 (1980).

Ahrentzen, S. B. (1990). Managing conflict by managing boundaries: How professional homeworkers cope with multiple roles at home. *Environment and Behavior, 22,* 723–752.

Ainsworth, M. (1978). *Patterns of attachment: A psychological study of the strange situation.* Hillsdale, NJ: Erlbaum.

American Association for Marriage and Family Therapists. (2001). *AAMFT code of ethics.* Alexandria, VA: Author. Retrieved July 8, 2001, from http://www.aamft.org/resources/LRMPlan/Ethics/ethicscode2001.asp

American Counseling Association. (2005). *ACA code of ethics.* Alexandria, VA: Author. Retrieved October 1, 2006, from http://www.counseling.org/Resources/CodeOfEthics/TP/Home/CT2.aspx

American Indian Mental Health Advisory Council. (2004). *Cultural competency guidelines for the provision of clinical mental health services to American Indians in the state of Minnesota.* Retrieved December 30, 2004, from http://edocs.dhs.state.mn.us/lfserver/Legacy/DHS-4086-ENG

American Psychiatric Association. (2001). *Principles of medical ethics with annotations especially applicable to psychiatry.* Washington, DC: Author. Retrieved June 9, 2003, from http://www.psych.org/apa_members/medicalethics2001_42001.cfm

American Psychological Association. (1953). *Ethical standards of psychologists.* Washington, DC: Author.

American Psychological Association. (1992). Ethical principles of psychologists and code of conduct. *American Psychologist, 47,* 1597–1611.

American Psychological Association. (1997). *Statement on services by telephone, teleconferencing, and Internet.* Retrieved July 1, 2005, from http://www.apa.org/ethics/stmnt01.html

American Psychological Association. (2002). Ethical principles of psychologists and code of conduct. *American Psychologist, 57,* 1060–1073. Retrieved October 4, 2006, from http://www.apa.org/ethics/code2002.html

Anderson, M. B., Van Raalte, L. L., & Brewer, B. W. (2001). Sports psychology service delivery: Staying ethical while keeping loose. *Professional Psychology: Research and Practice, 32,* 12–18.

Anderson, S. K., & Kitchener, K. S. (1998). Nonsexual post-therapy relationships: A conceptual framework to assess ethical risks. *Professional Psychology: Research and Practice, 29,* 91–99.

Aponte, J. F., & Wohl, J. (2000). *Psychological intervention and cultural diversity.* Boston: Allyn & Bacon.

Appelbaum, P. S. (1993). Legal liabilities and managed care. *American Psychologists, 48,* 251–257.

Aron, L. (1991). The patient's experience of the analyst's subjectivity. *Psychoanalytic Dialogues, 1,* 29–51.

Baer, B. E., & Murdock, N. L. (1995). Nonerotic dual relationships between therapist and clients: The effect of sex, theoretical orientation, and interpersonal boundaries. *Ethics and Behavior, 5,* 131–145.

Bailey, D. S. (2004, October) Approaching ethical dilemmas. *Monitor on Psychology, 35,* 62.

Banaka, W. H., & Young, D. W. (1985). Community coping skills enhanced by an adventure camp for adult chronic psychiatric patients. *Hospital and Community Psychiatry, 36,* 746–748.

Barnett, J. E. (1998). Should psychotherapists self-disclose? Clinical and ethical considerations. In L. VandeCreek, S. Knapp, & T. Jackson (Eds.), *Innovations in clinical practice: A source book* (Vol. 16, pp. 419–428). Sarasota, FL: Professional Resource Exchange.

Barnett, J. E. (1999). Multiple relationships: Ethical dilemmas and practical solutions. In L. VandeCreek, S. Knapp, & T. Jackson (Eds.), *Innovations in clinical practice: A source book* (Vol. 17, pp. 225–267). Sarasota, FL: Professional Resource Press.

Barnett, J. E., & Yutrzenka, B. A. (1994). Nonsexual dual relationships in professional practice, with special applications to rural and military communities. *The Independent Practitioner, 14,* 243–248.

Beauchamp, T. L., & Childress, J. F. (2001). *Principles of biomedical ethics* (5th ed.). New York: Oxford University Press.

Behnke, S. (2006, January). A letter to "Ethics Rounds." *Monitor on Psychology, 37,* 66.

Bennett, B. E., Bryant, B. K., VandenBos, G. R., & Greenwood, A. (1990). *Professional ability and risk management.* Washington, DC: American Psychological Association.

Berg, I. K. (1994). *Family-based services: A solution-focused approach.* New York: Norton.

Bernstein, A. C. (2000). Straight therapists working with lesbians and gays in family therapy. *Journal of Marriage and Family Therapy, 26,* 443–454.

Bersoff, D. (1999). *Ethical conflicts in psychology* (2nd ed.). Washington, DC: American Psychological Association.

Blanton, S. (1971). *Diary of my analysis with Sigmund Freud.* New York: Hawthorn Books.

Borys, D. S. (1992). Nonsexual dual relationships. In L. Vandecreek, S. Knapp, & T. L. Jackson (Eds.), *Innovations in clinical practice: A source book* (Vol. 11, pp. 443–454). Sarasota, FL: Professional Resource Exchange.

Borys, D. S., & Pope, K. S. (1989). Dual relationships between therapist and client: A national study of psychologists, psychiatrists, and social workers. *Professional Psychology: Research and Practice, 20,* 283–293.

Bowlby, J. (1969). *Attachment, separation and loss* (Vol. 1). New York: Basic Books.

Boyd-Franklin, N., & Bry, B. H. (2000). *Reaching out in family therapy: Home-based, school, and community interventions.* New York: Guilford Press.

Bridges, N. A. (2001). Therapist's self-disclosure: Expanding the comfort zone. *Psychotherapy, 38,* 21–30.

Brodsky, A. M. (1985). Sex between therapists and patients: Ethical gray areas. *Psychotherapy in Private Practice, 3*(1), 57–62.

Brown, L. S. (1984). The lesbian therapist in private practice and her community. *Psychotherapy in Private Practice, 2*(4), 9–16.

Brown, L. S. (1994). Boundaries in feminist therapy: A conceptual formulation. In N. K. Gartrell (Ed.), *Bringing ethics alive: Feminist ethics in psychotherapy practice* (pp. 29–38). New York: Haworth Press.

Bruce, M. L., & McNamara, R. (1992). Psychiatric status among the homebound elderly: An epidemiologic perspective. *Journal of American Geriatric Society, 40,* 561–566.

Bryce, M., & Lloyd, J. (Eds.). (1981). *Treating families in the home: An alternative to placement.* Springfield, IL: Charles C Thomas.

Bugental, J. F. (1987). *The art of the psychotherapist.* New York: Norton.

Burke, W. (1992). Countertransference disclosure and the asymmetry/mutuality dilemma. *Psychoanalytic Dialogue, 2,* 241–271.

Burns, D. D. (1990). *The feeling good handbook.* New York: Plume.

Bursten, B. (1959). The expressive value of gifts. *American Imago, 16,* 437–446.

Campbell, C. D., & Gordon, M. C. (2003). Acknowledging the inevitable: Understanding multiple relationships in rural practice. *Professional Psychology: Research and Practice, 34,* 430–434.

Canter, M., Bennett, B., Jones, S., & Nagy, T. (1996). *Ethics for psychologists.* Washington, DC: American Psychological Association.

Castelnuovo, G., Gaggioli, A., Mantovani, F., & Riva, G. (2003). New and old tools in psychotherapy and use of technology for the integration of traditional clinical treatments. *Psychotherapy: Theory, Research, Practice, Training, 40,* 1–2, 33–44.

Caudill, C. O. (2004). *Therapists under fire.* Retrieved June 1, 2004, from https://www.cphins.com/DesktopDefault.aspx?tabid=39

Cherniss, C., & Herzog, E. (1996). Impact of home-based family therapy on maternal and child outcomes in disadvantaged adolescent mothers. *Family Relations, 45,* 72–79.

Clark, S. C. (2000). Work/family border theory: A new theory of work/family balance. *Human Relations, 53,* 747–770.

Cohen, S. S. (1987). *The magic of touch.* New York: Harper & Row.

Cooper, S. (1998). Countertransference disclosure and the conceptualization of analytic technique. *Psychoanalytic Quarterly, 67,* 128–154.

Corey, G., Corey, M. S., & Callahan, P. (2003). *Issues and ethics in the helping professions* (6th ed.). Pacific Grove, CA: Brooks/Cole.

Cornell, W. F. (1997). Touch and boundaries in transactional analysis: Ethical and transferential considerations. *Transactional Analysis Journal, 37*(1), 30–37.

Cortes, L. (2004). Home-based family therapy: A misunderstanding of the role and a new challenge for therapists. *Family Journal, 12,* 184–188.

Cousins, N. (1985). Therapeutic value of laughter. *Integrative Psychiatry, 3,* 112.

Davis-Berman, J., & Berman, D. S. (1994). *Wilderness therapy: Foundations, theory and research.* Dubuque, IA: Kendall/Hunt.

DeJulio, L. M., & Berkman, C. S. (2003). Nonsexual multiple role relationships: Attitudes and behaviors of social workers. *Ethics and Behavior, 13,* 57–74.

Derrig-Palumbo, K., & Zeine, F. (2005). *Online therapy: A therapist's guide to expanding your practice.* New York: Norton.

Dineen, T. (1996). *Manufacturing victims: What the psychology industry is doing to people.* Westmount, Quebec, Canada: Robert Davies.

Doumanian, J. (Producer), & Allen, W. (Writer/Director). (1997). *Deconstructing Harry* [Motion picture]. United States: Jean Doumanian Productions and Sweetland Films.

Doverspike, W. F. (1999). *Ethical risk management: Guidelines for practice, a practical ethics handbook.* Sarasota, FL: Professional Resource Press.

Doverspike, W. F. (2004). Boundary violations and psychotherapy. *APA Review of Books, 49,* 209–211.

Downey, D. L. (2001). Therapeutic touch in psychotherapy. *Psychotherapy, 36*(1), 35–38.

Doyle, K. (1997). Substance abuse counselors in recovery: Implications for the ethical issues of dual relationships. *Journal of Counseling and Development, 75,* 428–432.

Dryden, W. (1990). Self-disclosure in rational emotive therapy. In G. Stricker & M. Fisher (Eds.), *Self-disclosure in the therapeutic relationship* (pp. 61–74). New York: Plenum Press.

Dunne, C., Bruggen, P., & O'Brien, C. (1982). Touch and action in group therapy of younger adolescents. *Journal of Adolescents, 5,* 31–38.

Durana, C. (1998). The use of touch in psychotherapy: Ethical and clinical guidelines. *Psychotherapy, 35,* 269–280.

Ebert, B. W. (1997). Dual-relationship prohibitions: A concept whose time never should have come. *Applied and Preventative Psychology, 6,* 137–156.

Epstein, R. S. (1994). *Keeping boundaries: Maintaining safety and integrity in the psychotherapeutic process.* Washington, DC: American Psychiatric Press.

Epstein, R. S., & Simon, R. I. (1990). The exploitation index: An early warning indicator of boundary violations in psychotherapy. *Bulletin of the Menninger Clinic, 54,* 450–465.

Epstein, R. S., Simon, R. I., & Kay, G. G. (1992). Assessing boundary violations in psychotherapy: Survey results with the exploitation index. *Bulletin of the Menninger Clinic, 56,* 150–166.

Erkolanhti, E., & Ilonen, T. (2004). A home-treatment system in child and adolescent psychiatry. *Clinical Child Psychology and Psychiatry, 9,* 427–436.

Ewert, A. (1987). Research in experiential education: An overview. *Journal of Experiential Education, 10*(2), 4–7.

Faulkner, K. K., & Faulkner, T. A. (1997). Managing multiple relationships in rural communities: Neutrality and boundary violations. *Clinical Psychology: Science and Practice, 4,* 225–234.

Faustman, W. O. (1982). Legal and ethical issues in debt collection strategies of professional psychologists. *Professional Psychology, 13,* 208–214.

Fay, A. (2002). The case against boundaries in psychotherapy. In A. A. Lazarus & O. Zur (Eds.), *Dual relationships and psychotherapy* (pp. 146–166). New York: Springer Publishing Company.

Feminist Therapy Institute. (1987). *Feminist therapy code of ethics.* Denver, CO: Author.

Field, T. (1998) Massage therapy effects. *American Psychologist, 53,* 1270–1281.

Fisher, C. D. (2004). Ethical issues in therapy: Therapist self-disclosure of sexual feelings. *Ethics and Behavior, 12,* 105–121.

Fosshage, J. L. (2000). The meanings of touch in psychoanalysis: A time for reassessment. *Psychoanalytic Inquiry, 20*(1). Retrieved July 1, 2004, from http://www.psychoanalyticinquiry.com/vol20no1.html

Frank, J. D. (1973). *Persuasion and healing: A comparative study of psychotherapy.* Baltimore: Johns Hopkins University Press.

Freeman, A., Fleming, B., & Pretzer, J. (1990). *Clinical applications of cognitive therapy.* New York: Plenum Press.

Fry, W., & Salameh, A. W. (1987). *Handbook of humor and psychotherapy.* Sarasota, FL: Professional Resource Press.

Gabbard, G. (Ed.). (1989). *Sexual exploitation in professional relationships.* Washington, DC: American Psychiatric Press.

Gabbard, G. (1994). Teetering on the precipice: A commentary on Lazarus's "How certain boundaries and ethics diminish therapeutic effectiveness." *Ethics and Behavior, 4,* 283–286.

Gabbard, G. O., & Lester, E. P. (1995). *Boundaries and boundary violations in psychoanalysis.* New York: Basic Books.

Gabbard, G. O., & Nadelson, C. (1995). Professional boundaries in the physician–patient relationship. *Journal of the American Medical Association, 273,* 1445–1449.

Gabbard, G. O., & Pope, K. S. (1989). Sexual intimacies after termination: Clinical, ethical, and legal aspects. In G. O. Gabbard (Ed.), *Sexual exploitation in professional relationships* (pp. 115–127). Washington, DC: American Psychiatric Press.

Gabriel, L. (2005). *Speaking the unspeakable: The ethics of dual relationships in counseling and psychotherapy.* New York: Routledge.

Gallagher, R. P., Gill, A. M., & Sysco, H. M. (2000). *National survey of counseling center directors 2000.* Alexandria, VA: International Association of Counseling Service.

Galloway, G., & Cropley, A. (1999). Benefits of humor for mental health: Empirical findings and directions for further research. *International Journal of Humor Research, 12,* 301–314.

Gass, M. A. (1993). *Adventure therapy: Therapeutic applications of adventure programming.* Dubuque, IA: Kendall/Hunt.

Gerson, A., & Fox, D. D. (1999). Boundary violations: The gray area. *American Journal of Forensic Psychology, 17*(2), 57–61.

Geyer, M. C. (1994). Dual role relationships and Christian counseling. *Journal of Psychology and Theology, 22,* 187–195.

Glass, J. S., & Shoffner, M. F. (2001). Adventure-based counseling in schools. *Professional School Counseling, 5,* 42–47.

Glover, E. (1940). *An investigation of the technique of psychoanalysis.* Baltimore: Williams & Wilkins.

Gody, D. S. (1996). Chance encounters: Unintentional therapist disclosure. *Psychoanalytic Psychology, 13,* 495–511.

Goldfried, M. R., Burckell, L. A., & Eubanks-Carter, C. (2003). Therapist self-disclosure in cognitive–behavior therapy. *Journal of Clinical Psychology, 59,* 555–568.

Goldstein, E. G. (1997). To tell or not to tell: The disclosure of events in the therapist's life to the patient. *Clinical Social Work Journal, 25,* 41–58.

Gonsiorek, J. C., & Brown, L. S. (1989). Post therapy sexual relationships with clients. In G. R. Schoener, J. H. Milgrom, J. C. Gonsiorek, E. T. Luepker, & R. M. Conroe (Eds.), *Psychotherapists' sexual involvement with clients: Intervention and prevention* (pp. 289–301). Minneapolis, MN: Walk-in Counseling Center.

Gottlieb, M. C. (1993). Avoiding exploitative dual relationships: A decision-making model. *Psychotherapy, 30,* 41–48.

Grayson, P. A. (1986). Mental health confidentiality on the small campus. *Journal of American College Health, 34,* 187–191.

Greenspan, M. (1986). Should therapists be personal? Self-disclosure and therapeutic distance in feminist therapy. In D. Howard (Ed.), *The dynamics of feminist therapy* (pp. 5–17). New York: Haworth Press.

Greenspan, M. (1995, July/August). Out of bounds. *Common Boundary Magazine,* 51–56.

Grohol, J. M. (1999). *Best practices in e-therapy: Definition and scope of e-therapy.* Retrieved April 5, 2005, from http://psychcentral.com/best/best3.htm

Grosskurth, P. (1991). *The secret ring: Freud's inner circle and the politics of psychoanalysis.* Toronto, Ontario, Canada: Macfarlane Walter & Ross.

Gutheil, T. G. (1989, November/December). Patient–therapist sexual relations. *The California Therapist,* 29–39.

Gutheil, T. G. (1998). *The psychiatrist as expert witness.* Washington, DC: American Psychiatric Press.

Gutheil, T. G., & Gabbard, G. O. (1993). The concept of boundaries in clinical practice: Theoretical and risk-management dimensions. *American Journal of Psychiatry, 150,* 188–196.

Gutheil, T. G., & Gabbard, G. O. (1998). Misuses and misunderstandings of boundary theory in clinical and regulatory settings. *American Journal of Psychiatry, 155,* 409–414.

Guthmann, D., & Sandberg, K. A. (2002). Dual relationships in the deaf community: When dual relationships are unavoidable and essential. In A. A. Lazarus & O. Zur (Eds.), *Dual relationships and psychotherapy* (pp. 287–297). New York: Springer Publishing Company.

Haas, L. J., & Malouf, J. L. (1989). *Keeping up the good work: A practitioner's guide to mental health ethics.* Sarasota, FL: Professional Resource Exchange.

Hahn, W. K. (1998). Gifts in psychotherapy: An intersubjective approach to patient gifts. *Psychotherapy: Theory, Research, Practice, Training, 35,* 78–86.

Halbrook, B., & Duplechin, R. (1994). Rethinking touch in psychotherapy: Guidelines for practitioners. *Psychotherapy in Private Practice, 13*(3), 43–53.

Hanson, J. E. (2003). *Coming out: Therapist self-disclosure as a therapeutic technique, with specific application to sexual minority populations.* Retrieved January 10, 2005, from http://www.oise.utoronto.ca/depts/aecp/CMPConf/papers/Hanson.html

Hargrove, D. S. (1986). Ethical issues in rural mental health practice. *Professional Psychology: Research and Practice, 17,* 20–23.

Harlow, H. (1971). *Learning to love.* New York: Albion.

Harris, S. R. (2002). Dual relationships and university counseling center environments. In A. A. Lazarus & O. Zur (Eds.), *Dual relationships and psychotherapy* (pp. 337–347). New York: Springer Publishing Company.

Hayman, P. M., & Cover, J. A. (1986). Ethical dilemmas in college counseling centers. *Journal of Counseling and Development, 64,* 318–320.

Health Insurance Portability and Accountability Act of 1996, 104th Cong., Pub. L. No. 104-191.

Heath, D. S. (2005). *Home treatments for acute mental disorders: An alternative to hospitalization.* New York: Routledge.

Hedges, L. E., Hilton, R., Hilton, V. W., & Caudill, O. B. (1997). *Therapists at risk: Perils of the intimacy of the therapeutic relationships.* Northvale, NJ.

Helbok, C. M. (2003). The practice of psychology in rural communities: Potential ethical dilemmas. *Ethics and Behavior, 13,* 367–384.

Helbok, C. M., Marinelli, R. P., & Walls, R. T. (2006). National survey of ethical practices across rural and urban communities. *Professional Psychology: Research and Practice, 37,* 36–44.

Heller, S. (1997). *The vital touch.* New York: Holt.

Herbert, J. T. (1996). Use of adventure-based counseling programs for persons with disabilities. *Journal of Rehabilitation, 62,* 3–9.

Herlihy, B., & Corey, G. (2006). *Boundary issues in counseling: Multiple roles and responsibilities* (2nd ed.). Alexandria, VA: American Association for Counseling and Development.

Hill, M. (1999). Barter: Ethical considerations in psychotherapy. *Women and Therapy, 22*(3), 81–91.

Hines, A. H., Adler, D. N., Chang, A. S., & Rundell, J. R. (1998). Dual agency, dual relationships, boundary crossings, and associated boundary violations: A survey of military and civilian psychiatrists. *Military Medicine, 163,* 826–833.

Hollinger, L. (1986). Communicating with the elderly. *Journal of Gerontological Nursing, 12*(3), 8–13.

Holroyd, J. C., & Brodsky, A. (1980). Does touching patients lead to sexual intercourse? *Professional Psychology, 11,* 807–811.

Holub, E. A., & Lee, S. S. (1990). Therapists' use of nonerotic physical contact: Ethical concerns. *Professional Psychology: Research and Practice, 21,* 115–117.

Horton, J., Clance, P. R., Sterk-Elifson, C., & Emshoff, J. (1995). Touch in psychotherapy: A survey of patients' experiences. *Psychotherapy, 32,* 443–457.

Hunter, M., & Struve, J. (1998). *The ethical use of touch in psychotherapy.* Thousand Oaks, CA: Sage.

Hyman, S. M. (2002). The shirtless jock therapist and the bikini-clad client: An exploration of chance extra-therapeutic encounters. In A. A. Lazarus &

O. Zur (Eds.), *Dual relationships and psychotherapy* (pp. 348–359). New York: Springer Publishing Company.

Isaac, T. (2004). Ethical notes on disrupted frames and violated boundaries. *Psychoanalytic Psychology, 21,* 609–613.

Isay, R. A. (1996). *Becoming gay: The journey to self-acceptance.* New York: Holt.

Johnson, W. B. (1995). Perennial ethical quandaries in military psychology: Toward American Psychological Association and Department of Defense collaboration. *Professional Psychology: Research and Practice, 26,* 281–287.

Johnson, W. B., Ralph, J., & Johnson, S. J. (2005). Managing multiple roles in embedded environments: The case of aircraft carrier psychology. *Professional Psychology: Research and Practice, 36,* 73–81.

Johnston, S. H., & Farber, B. A. (1996). The maintenance of boundaries in psychotherapeutic practice. *Psychotherapy, 33,* 391–402.

Jones, E. (1957). *The life and work of Sigmund Freud: Vol. III. The last phase, 1919–1939.* New York: Basic Books.

Jones, M., Botsko, M., & Gorman, B. S. (2003). Predictors of psychotherapeutic benefit of lesbian, gay, and bisexual clients: The effects of sexual orientation matching and other factors. *Psychotherapy: Theory, Research, Practice, Training, 40,* 289–301.

Jourard, S. M. (1971a). *Self-disclosure: An experimental analysis of the transparent self.* New York: Wiley-Interscience.

Jourard, S. M. (1971b). *The transparent self.* New York: Van Nostrand Reinhold.

Kanter, R. M. (1977). *Work and family in the United States: A critical review and agenda for research and policy.* New York: Russell Foundation.

Kerr, J. (1993). *A most dangerous method.* New York: Knopf.

Kertész, R. (2002). Dual relationships in psychotherapy in Latin America. In A. A. Lazarus & O. Zur (Eds.), *Dual relationships and psychotherapy* (pp. 329–334). New York: Springer Publishing Company.

Kessler, L. E., & Waehler, C. A. (2005). Ethical issues in professional practice: Addressing multiple relationships between clients and therapists in lesbian, gay, bisexual, and transgender communities. *Professional Psychology: Research and Practice, 36,* 66–72.

Kitchener, K. S. (1988). Dual role relationships: What makes them so problematic? *Journal of Counseling and Development, 67,* 217–221.

Knapp, M. L., & Hall, J. A. (1997). *Nonverbal communication in human interaction* (4th ed.). Fort Worth, TX: Harcourt Brace.

Knapp, S. J., & Slattery, J. M. (2004). Professional boundaries in nontraditional settings. *Professional Psychology: Research and Practice, 14,* 553–558.

Knapp, S. J., & VandeCreek, L. D. (2006). *Practical ethics for psychologists: A positive approach.* Washington, DC: American Psychological Association.

Knox, S., Hess, S. A., Petersen, D. A., & Hill, C. E. (1997). A qualitative analysis of client perceptions of the effects of helpful therapist self-disclosure in long-term therapy. *Journal of Counseling Psychology, 44,* 274–283.

Knox, S., Hess, S. A., Williams, E. N., & Hill, C. E. (2003). Here's a little something for you: How therapists respond to clients' gifts. *Journal of Counseling Psychology, 50,* 199–210.

Kohn, R., Phil, M., Goldsmith, E., & Sedgwick, T. W. (2002). Treatment of homebound mentally ill elderly patients: The multidisciplinary psychiatric mobile team. *American Journal of Geriatric Psychiatry, 10,* 469–475.

Koocher, G. P., & Keith-Spiegel, P. (1998). *Ethics in psychology: Professional standards and cases* (2nd ed.). New York: Oxford University Press.

Koocher, G. P., & Morray, E. (2000). Regulation of telepsychology: A survey of state attorneys general. *Professional Psychology: Research and Practice, 31,* 503–508.

Kossek, E. (2003). *Setting boundaries between work and life helps families thrive.* Retrieved May 8, 2003, from http://newsroom.msu.edu/site/indexer/1433/content.htm

Kritzberg, N. I. (1980). On patients' gift-giving. *Contemporary Psychoanalysis, 16,* 98–118.

Lakin, M. (1991). *Coping with ethical dilemmas in psychotherapy.* New York: Pergamon Press.

Lally, M. C., & Freeman, S. A. (2005). The struggle to maintain neutrality in the treatment of patients with pedophilia. *Ethics and Behavior, 15,* 182–190.

Lamb, D. H., & Catanzaro, S. J. (1998). Sexual and nonsexual boundary violations involving psychologists, clients, supervisees, and students: Implications for professional practice. *Professional Psychology: Research and Practice, 29,* 498–503.

Lamb, D. H., Catanzaro, S. J., & Moorman, A. S. (2004). A preliminary look at how psychologists identify, evaluate, and proceed when faced with possible multiple relationship dilemmas. *Professional Psychology: Research and Practice, 35,* 248–254.

Lamb, M. E., Thompson, W., Gardner, & Charnov, E. L. (1985). *Infant–mother attachment: The origins and developmental significance of individual differences in strange situation behavior.* Hillside, NJ: Erlbaum.

Lambert, M. J. (1991). Introduction to psychotherapy research. In L. E. Beutler & M. Cargo (Eds.), *Psychotherapy research: An international review of programmatic studies* (pp. 1–11). Washington, DC: American Psychological Association.

Langs, R. (1982). *Psychotherapy: A basic text.* New York: Aronson.

Lawry, S. (1998). Touch and clients who have been sexually abused. In M. Hunter & J. Struve (Eds.), *The ethical use of touch in psychotherapy* (pp. 201–210). New York: Guilford Press.

Lazarus, A. A. (1994). How certain boundaries and ethics diminish therapeutic effectiveness. *Ethics and Behavior, 4,* 255–261.

Lazarus, A. A. (1998). How do you like these boundaries? *The Clinical Psychologist, 51,* 22–25.

Lazarus, A. A., & Zur, O. (2002). *Dual relationships and psychotherapy.* New York: Springer Publishing Company.

Lemma, A. (1999). *Humour on the couch: Exploring humour in psychotherapy and everyday life.* London: Whurr.

Lewis, P. (1959). A note on the private aspect of the psychoanalyst. *Bulletin of the Philadelphia Psychoanalytic Association, 9,* 96–101.

Liddle, B. J. (1997). Gay and lesbian clients' selection of therapists and utilization of therapy. *Psychotherapy, 34,* 11–18.

Little, M. I. (1990). *Psychotic anxieties and containment: A personal record of an analysis with Winnicott.* Northvale, NJ: Aronson.

Llewellyn, R. (2002). Sanity and sanctity: The counselor and multiple relationships in the church. In A. A. Lazarus & O. Zur (Eds.), *Dual relationships and psychotherapy* (pp. 298–314). New York: Springer Publishing Company.

Lowen, A. (1976). *Bioenergetics.* New York: Penguin.

Lowry, T. (1974). *Camping therapy: Its uses in psychiatry and rehabilitation.* Springfield, IL: Charles C Thomas.

MacHovec, F. (1991). Humor in therapy. *Psychotherapy in Private Practice, 9,* 25–33.

Maeder, T. (1989). *Children of psychiatrists and other psychotherapists.* New York: Harper & Row.

Mahalik, J. R., van Ormer, E. A., & Simi, N. L. (2000). Ethical issues in using self-disclosure in feminist therapy. In M. M. Brabeck (Ed.), *Practicing feminist ethics in psychology* (pp. 189–201). Washington, DC: American Psychological Association.

Maheu, M. M., & Gordon, B. L. (2000). Counseling and therapy on the Internet. *Professional Psychology: Research and Practice, 31,* 484–489.

Maheu, M. M., Pulier, M. L., Wilhelm, F. H., McMenamin, J. P., & Brown-Connolly, N. E. (2005). *The mental health professional and the new technologies: A handbook for practice today.* Mahwah, NJ: Erlbaum.

Maheu, M., Whitten, P., & Allen, A. (2001). *E-health, telehealth, and telemedicine: A guide to startup and success.* New York: Jossey-Bass.

Mallow, A. J. (1998). Self-disclosure: Reconciling psychoanalytic psychotherapy and Alcoholics Anonymous philosophy. *Journal of Substance Abuse Treatment, 15,* 493–498.

McDermott, D., Tyndall, L., & Lichtenberg, J. W. (1989). Factors related to counselor preference among gays and lesbians. *Journal of Counseling and Development, 68,* 31–35.

Mehrabian, A. (1971). *The silent language: Implicit communication of emotions and attitudes.* Belmont, CA: Wadsworth.

Menikoff, A. (1999). *Psychiatric home care: Clinical and economic dimensions.* New York: Academic Press.

Menninger, K. (1958*). Theory of psychoanalytic technique.* New York: Basic Books.

Milakovitch, J. C. (1993). Touching in psychotherapy: The differences between therapists who touch and those who do not. *Dissertation Abstracts International, 54*(6-B), 334.

Minuchin, S. (1974). *Families and family therapy.* Cambridge, MA: Harvard University Press.

Moleski, S. M., & Kiselica, M. S. (2005). Dual relationships: A continuum ranging from destructive to therapeutic. *Journal of Counseling and Development, 83*, 3–11.

Montagu, A. (1971). *Touching: The human significance of the skin.* New York: Columbia University Press.

Montgomery, M. J., & DeBell, C. (1997). Dual relationships and pastoral counseling: Asset or liability? *Counseling and Values, 42*, 30–41.

Moore, Z. E. (2003). Ethical dilemmas in sport psychology: Discussion and recommendation for practice. *Professional Psychology: Research and Practice, 34*, 601–610.

Morris, J. (2003). The home visit in family therapy. *Journal of Family Psychotherapy, 14*, 95–99.

Nagy, T. F. (2005). *Ethics in plain English: An illustrative casebook for psychologists* (2nd ed.). Washington, DC: American Psychological Association.

National Association of Social Workers. (1996). *NASW code of ethics.* Washington, DC: Author.

National Association of Social Workers. (1999). *Code of ethics.* Retrieved July 27, 2001, from http://www.socialworkers.org/pubs/code/code.asp

National Board for Certified Counselors. (2005a). *National Board for Certified Counselors code of ethics.* Retrieved July 27, 2006, from http://www.nbcc.org/extras/pdfs/ethics/nbcc-codeofethics.pdf

National Board for Certified Counselors. (2005b). *The practice of Internet counseling.* Retrieved August 28, 2006, from http://www.nbcc.org/webethics2

Nickel, M. (2004). Professional boundaries: The dilemma of dual and multiple relationships in rural clinical practice. *Consulting and Clinical Psychology Journal, 1*, 17–22.

Norcross, J. C., & Goldfried, M. R. (Eds.). (1992). *Handbook of psychotherapy integration.* New York: Basic Books.

Nordmarken, N., & Zur, O. (2004). *To touch or not to touch: Rethinking the prohibition on touch in psychotherapy and counseling: Clinical, ethical and legal consid-*

erations. Retrieved August 5, 2005, from http://www.drzur.com/touchintherapy.html

Nordmarken, N., & Zur, O. (2005). *Home office: Ethical and clinical considerations.* Retrieved August 8, 2005, from http://www.drzur.com/homeoffice.html

Older, J. (1982). *Touching is healing.* New York: Stein & Day.

Oz, F. (Director), Sargent, A. (Writer), Ziskin, L. (Writer), & Schulman, T. (Screenplay). (1991). *What about Bob?* [Motion picture]. United States: Touchstone Pictures.

Pedersen, P. B., Draguns, J. G., Lonner, W. J., & Trimble, J. E. (Eds.). (1996). *Counseling across cultures.* (4th ed.). Thousand Oaks, CA: Sage.

Pepper, R. S. (1990). When transference isn't transference: Iatrogenesis of multiple role relations between practicing therapists. *Journal of Contemporary Psychotherapy, 20,* 141–153.

Pepper, R. S. (2003). Be it ever so humble: The controversial issue of psychotherapy groups in the home office setting. *Groups, 27*(1), 41–52.

Perlmutter, M. S., & Hatfield, E. (1980). Intimacy, intentional metacommunication and second order change. *American Journal of Family Therapy, 8,* 17–23.

Perls, F. (1973). *The Gestalt approach and eye witness to therapy.* Palo Alto, CA: Science & Behavior Books.

Peterson, C. (1996). Common problem areas and their causes resulting in disciplinary action. In L. J. Bass, S. T. DeMers, J. R. P. Ogloff, C. Peterson, J. L. Pettifor, R. P. Reaves, et al. (Eds.), *Professional conduct and discipline in psychology* (pp. 71–89). Washington, DC: American Psychological Association.

Peterson, Z. D. (2002). More than a mirror: The ethics of therapist self-disclosure. *Psychotherapy: Theory, Research, Practice, Training, 19,* 21–31.

Polster, D. S. (2001). *Gifts: American Psychiatric Association ethics primer.* Washington, DC: American Psychiatric Press.

Pope, K. S. (1989). Therapist–patient sex syndrome: A guide to assessing damage. In G. O. Gabbard (Ed.), *Sexual exploitation in professional relationships* (pp. 39–55). Washington, DC: American Psychiatric Press.

Pope, K. S. (1990a). Therapist–patient sex as sex abuse: Six scientific, professional, and practical dilemmas in addressing victimization and rehabilitation. *Professional Psychology: Research and Practice, 21,* 227–239.

Pope, K. S. (1990b). Therapist–patient esexual contact: Clinical, legal, and ethical implications. In E. A. Margenau, *The encyclopedia handbook of private practice* (pp. 687–696). New York: Gardner Press.

Pope, K. S., Keith-Spiegel, P., & Tabachnick, B. G. (1986). Sexual attraction to clients: The human therapist and the (sometimes) inhuman training system. *American Psychologist, 41,* 147–158.

Pope, K. S., Sonne, J., & Holroyd, J. (1993). *Sexual feelings in psychotherapy: Exploration for therapists and therapists-in-training*. Washington, DC: American Psychological Association.

Pope, K. S., Tabachnick, B. G., & Keith-Spiegel, K. (1987). Ethics of practice: The beliefs and behaviors of psychologists as therapists. *American Psychologist, 42*, 993–1006.

Pope, K. S., & Vasquez, M. J. T. (2001). *Ethics in psychotherapy and counseling: A practical guide* (2nd ed.). San Francisco: Jossey-Bass.

Prescott, J. W. (1975, April). Bodly pleasure and the origins of violence. *The Futurist, April*, 64–67.

Psychopathology Committee of the Group for the Advancement of Psychiatry. (2001). Reexamination of therapist self-disclosure. *Psychiatric Services, 52*, 1489–1493.

Pulakos, J. (1994). Incidental encounters between therapists and clients: The client's perspective. *Professional Psychology, 25*, 300–303.

Ramsdell, P. S., & Ramsdell, E. R. (1993). Dual relationships: Client perceptions of the effect of client–counselor relationship on the therapeutic process. *Clinical Social Work Journal, 21*, 195–212.

Rappoport, S. P. (1983). *Value for value psychotherapy: The economic and therapeutic barter*. New York: Praeger Publishers.

Reamer, F. G. (2001). *Tangled relationships: Managing boundary issues in human services*. New York: Columbia University Press.

Recupero, P. R. (2005). E-mail and the psychiatrist–patient relationship. *Journal of American Academy of Psychiatry and Law, 33*, 465–475.

Redford, R. (Director). (1980). *Ordinary people* [Motion picture]. United States: Paramount Pictures and Wildwood Enterprises.

Rees, C. S., & Stone, S. (2005). Therapeutic alliance in face-to-face versus videoconferenced psychotherapy. *Professional Psychology: Research and Practice, 36*, 649–653.

Reich, W. (1972). *Character analysis*. New York: Simon & Schuster.

Reist, D., & VandeCreek, L. (2004). The pharmaceutical industry's use of gifts and educational events to influence prescription practices: Ethical dilemmas and implications for psychologists. *Professional Psychology: Research and Practice, 35*, 329–335.

Renik, O. (1996). The ideal of the anonymous analyst and the problem of self-disclosure. *Psychoanalytic Quarterly, 65*, 681–682.

Roberts, R. N., Wasik, B. H., Casto, G., & Ramey, C. T. (1991). Family support in the home: Programs, policy, and social change. *American Psychologist, 46*, 131–137.

Rogers, C. (1970). *Carl Rogers on encounter groups*. New York: Harper & Row.

Rosen, L. D., & Weill, M. M. (1997). *The mental health technology bible.* New York: Wiley.

Rosie, J. S. (1974). The therapists' self-disclosure in individual psychotherapy: Research and psychoanalytic theory. *Journal of Consulting and Clinical Psychology, 42,* 901–908.

Rueveni, U. (1979). *Networking families in crisis: Intervention strategies with families and social networks.* New York: Human Sciences Library.

Rutter, P. (1989). *Sex in the forbidden zone: When men in power—therapists, doctors, clergy, teachers, and others—betray women's trust.* New York: Fawcett Crest.

Saad, G., & Gill, T. (2003). An evolutionary psychology perspective on gift-giving among young adults. *Psychology and Marketing, 20,* 765–784.

Satir, V. (1972). *Peoplemaking.* Palo Alto, CA: Science & Behavior Books.

Schacht, A. J., Tafoya, N., & Mirabla, K. (1989). Home-based therapy with American Indian families. *American Indian and Alaska Native Mental Health Research, 3*(2), 27–42.

Schank, A. J., & Skovholt, T. M. (1997). Dual-relationship dilemmas of rural and small-community psychologists. *Professional Psychology: Research and Practice, 28,* 44–49.

Schank, A. J., & Skovholt, T. M. (2006). *Ethical practice in small communities: Challenges and rewards for psychologists.* Washington, DC: American Psychological Association.

Schoel, J., Prouty, D., & Radcliffe, P. (1988). *Islands of healing: A guide to adventure based counseling.* Hamilton, MA: Project Adventure.

Schoener, G. R. (1997, September). *Boundaries in professional relationships.* Paper presented at the meeting of the Norwegian Psychological Association, Oslo, Norway.

Schultz, L. G. (1975). A survey of social workers' attitudes and use of body and sex psychotherapies. *Clinical Social Work Journal, 3,* 90–99.

Schwartz, M. D. (1975). Casework implications of a worker's pregnancy. *Social Casework, 56,* 27–34.

Sears, V. L. (1990). On being an "only" one. In H. Lerman & N. Porter (Eds.), *Feminist ethics in psychotherapy* (pp. 102–105). New York: Springer Publishing Company.

Shapiro, E. L., & Ginzberg, R. (2003). To accept or not to accept: Referrals and the maintenance of boundaries. *Professional Psychology: Research and Practice, 34,* 258–263.

Sharkin, B. (1995). Strains on confidentiality in college-student psychotherapy: Entangled therapeutic relationships, incidental encounters, and third-party inquiries. *Professional Psychology: Research and Practice, 26,* 184–189.

Sharkin, B. S., & Birky, I. (1992). Incidental encounters between therapists and their clients. *Professional Psychology: Research and Practice, 23,* 326–328.

Silber, A. (1969). A patient's gift: Its meaning and function. *International Journal of Psychoanalysis, 50,* 335–341.

Simi, N. L., & Mahalik, J. R. (1997). Comparison of feminist versus psychoanalytic/dynamic and other therapists on self-disclosure. *Psychology of Women Quarterly, 21,* 465–483.

Simon, R. I. (1991). Psychological injury caused by boundary violation: Precursors to therapist–patient sex. *Psychiatric Annals, 21,* 614–619.

Simon, R. I. (1994). Transference in therapist–patient sex: The illusion of patient improvement and consent, Part 1. *Psychiatric Annals, 24,* 509–515.

Simon, R. I., & Williams, I. C. (1999). Maintaining treatment boundaries in small communities and rural areas. *Psychiatric services, 50,* 1440–1446.

Slattery, J. M. (2005). Preventing role slippage during work in the community: Guidelines for new psychologists and supervisees. *Psychotherapy: Theory, Research, Practice, Training, 42,* 384–394.

Sleek, S. (1994, December). Ethical dilemmas plague rural practice. *Monitor on Psychology,* 25–26.

Smith, A. J. (1990). Working within the lesbian community: The dilemma of overlapping relationships. In H. Lerman & N. Porter (Eds.), *Feminist ethics in psychotherapy* (pp. 92–96). New York: Springer Publishing Company.

Smith, D., & Fitzpatrick, M. (1995). Patient–therapist boundary issues: An integrative review of theory and research. *Professional Psychology: Research and Practice, 25,* 499–506.

Smith, E., Clance, P .R., & Imes, S. (Eds.). (1998). *Touch in psychotherapy: Theory, research and practice.* New York: Guilford Press.

Smolar, A. M. (2003). When we give more: Reflections on intangible gifts from therapist to patient. *American Journal of Psychotherapy, 57,* 300–323.

Snyder, W., & McCollum, E. E. (1999). Their home is their castle: Learning to do in-home family therapy. *Family Process, 38,* 229–242.

Sonne, J. L. (1994). Multiple relationships: Does the new ethics code answer the right questions? *Professional Psychology: Research and Practice, 25,* 331–343.

Sonne, J. L., & Pope, K. S. (1991). Treating victims of therapist–patient involvement. *Psychotherapy, 28,* 174–187.

Spandler, H., Burman, E., Goldberg, B., Margison, F., & Amos, T. (2000). A double edged sword: Understanding gifts in psychotherapy. *European Journal of Psychotherapy, Counseling and Health, 3*(1), 77–101.

St. Germaine, J. (1996). Dual relationships and certified alcohol and drug counselors: A national study of ethical beliefs and behaviors. *Alcoholism Treatment Quarterly, 14*(2), 29–45.

Staal, M. A., & King, R. E. (2000). Managing a multiple relationship environment: The ethics of military psychology. *Professional Psychology: Research and Practice, 31,* 698–705.

Stamm, B. H. (1998). Clinical applications of telehealth in mental health care. *Professional Psychology: Research and Practice, 29,* 536–542.

Stamm, B. H. (2003). *Rural behavioral health care: An interdisciplinary guide.* Washington, DC: American Psychological Association.

Stein, H. (1965). The gift in therapy. *American Journal of Psychotherapy, 19,* 480–486.

Sterling, D. L. (1992). Practicing rural psychotherapy: Complexity of role and boundary. *Psychotherapy in Private Practice, 10,* 105–127.

Stockman, A. F. (1990). Dual relationships in rural mental health practice: An ethical dilemma. *Journal of Rural Community Psychology, 11,* 31–45.

Strasburger, L. H., Jorgenson, L., & Sutherland, P. (1992). The prevention of psychotherapist sexual misconduct: Avoiding the slippery slope. *American Journal of Psychotherapy, 46,* 544–555.

Strean, H. S. (1981). Extra-analytic contacts: Theoretical and clinical considerations. *Psychoanalytic Quarterly, 56,* 238–257.

Stricker, G., & Fisher, M. (Eds.). (1990). *Self-disclosure in the therapeutic relationship.* New York: Plenum Press.

Sue, D., & Sue, D. (2003). *Counseling the culturally diverse: Theory and practice* (4th ed.). New York: Wiley.

Syme, G. (2003). *Dual relationships in counseling and psychotherapy: Exploring the limit.* London: Sage.

Tabachnick, B. G., Keith-Spiegel, P. C., & Pope, K. S. (1991). Ethics of teaching: Beliefs and behaviors of psychologists as educators. *American Psychologist, 46,* 506–515.

Talan, K. H. (1989). Gifts in psychoanalysis. *Psychoanalytic Study of the Child, 44,* 149–163.

Tantillo, M. M. (2004). The therapist's use of self-disclosure in a relational therapy approach for eating disorders. *Eating Disorders, 12*(1), 51–73.

Tarnower, W. (1966). Extra-analytic contacts between the psychoanalyst and the patient. *Psychoanalytic Quarterly, 35,* 399–413.

Telehealth Improvement and Modernization Act of 2000, S. 2505.IS.

Thomas, J. L. (2002). Bartering. In A. A. Lazarus & O. Zur (Eds.), *Dual relationships and psychotherapy* (pp. 394–408). New York: Springer Publishing Company.

Tillman, J. G. (1998). Psychodynamic psychotherapy, religious beliefs, and self-disclosure. *Journal of Psychotherapy, 52,* 273–286.

Tirnauer, L., Smith, E., & Foster, P. (1996). The American Academy of Psychotherapists research committee survey of members. *Voices, 32*(2), 87–94.

Tomm, K. (1993). The ethics of dual relationships. *California Therapist, 5*(1), 7–19.

Trimble, J. E. (2002). *Counseling across cultures.* Thousand Oaks, CA: Sage.

U.S. Association for Body Psychotherapy. (2001). *Ethics guidelines*. Bethesda, MD: Author. Retrieved July 1, 2005, from http://www.usabp.org/associations/1808/files/USABPethics.pdf

U.S. Department of Health and Human Services. (1999). *Mental health: A report of the Surgeon General, executive summary*. Rockville, MD: Author.

Van Sant, G. (Director), Damon, M. (Writer), & Affleck, B. (Writer). (1997). *Good Will Hunting* [Motion picture]. United States: Miramax Films.

VandenBos, G. R., & Williams, S. (2000). The Internet versus the telephone: What is telehealth, anyway? *Professional Psychology: Research and Practice, 31*, 490–492.

Vinogradov, S., & Yalom, I. D. (1990). Self-disclosure in group psychotherapy. In G. Stricker & M. Fisher (Eds.), *Self-disclosure in the therapeutic relationship* (pp. 191–204). New York: Plenum Press.

Volker, T. (1999). Beyond the clinic: In-home therapy with Head Start families. *Journal of Marital and Family Therapy, 25*, 177–189.

Wakefield, J. (1996). *Dual-role relationships in training*. Retrieved March 9, 2001, from http://www.cgjungpage.org/articles/jwake1.html

Welfel, E. R. (2002). *Ethics in counseling and psychotherapy: Standards, research, and emerging issues* (2nd ed.). Pacific Grove, CA: Brooks/Cole.

White, M., & Epston, D. (1990). *Narrative means to therapeutic ends*. New York: Norton.

Williams, M. H. (1997). Boundary violations: Do some contended standards of care fail to encompass commonplace procedures of humanistic, behavioral, and eclectic psychotherapies? *Psychotherapy, 34*, 238–249.

Williams, M. H. (2002). Multiple relationships: A malpractice plaintiffs' litigation strategy. In A. A. Lazarus & O. Zur (Eds.), *Dual relationships and psychotherapy* (pp. 228–238). New York: Springer Publishing Company.

Williams, M. H. (2003). The curse of risk management. *The Independent Practitioner, 23*, 202–205.

Wolberg, L. (1967). *The technique of psychotherapy* (2nd ed.). New York: Grune & Stratton.

Woody, R. H. (1988). *Protecting your mental health practice: How to minimize legal and financial risk*. San Francisco: Jossey-Bass.

Woody, R. H. (1998). Bartering for psychological services. *Professional Psychology: Research and Practice, 29*, 174–178.

Woody R. H. (1999). Domestic violations of confidentiality. *Professional Psychology: Research and Practice, 30*, 607–610.

Yalom, I. D. (1975). *The theory and practice of group psychotherapy*. New York: Basic Books.

Yalom, I. D., & Elkin, G. (1990). *Every day gets a little closer: A twice-told therapy*. New York: Basic Books.

Younggren, J. N., & Gottlieb, M. C. (2004). Managing risk when contemplating multiple relationships. *Professional Psychology: Research and Practice, 35,* 255–260.

Zelig, M. (1988). Ethical dilemmas in police psychology. *Professional Psychology: Research and Practice, 19,* 336–338.

Zimbardo, P. G. (2004). Does psychology make a significant difference in our lives? *American Psychologist, 59,* 339–351.

Zur, O. (2000). In celebration of dual relationships: How prohibition of non-sexual dual relationships increases the chance of exploitation and harm. *The Independent Practitioner, 2*(3), 97–100.

Zur, O. (2001a). On analysis, transference and dual relationships: A rejoinder to Dr. Pepper. *The Independent Practitioner, 21*(3), 201–204.

Zur, O. (2001b). Out-of-office experience: When crossing office boundaries and engaging in dual relationships are clinically beneficial and ethically sound. *The Independent Practitioner, 21*(1), 96–100.

Zur, O. (2004a). A chicken for a session: Bartering in therapy. *Voices, 40*(1), 75–80.

Zur, O. (2004b). To cross or not to cross: Do boundaries in therapy protect or harm? *Psychotherapy Bulletin, 39*(3), 27–32.

Zur, O. (2005a). Dumbing down of psychology: Manufactured consent about the depravity of dual relationships in therapy. In R. H. Wright & N. A. Cummings (Eds.), *Destructive trends in mental health: The well-intentioned road to harm* (pp. 253–282). New York: Brunner-Routledge.

Zur, O. (2005b). *HIPAA compliance kit* (3rd ed.). Sonoma, CA: OZ Books.

Zur, O., & Gonzalez, S. (2002). Multiple relationships in military psychology. In A. A. Lazarus & O. Zur (Eds.), *Dual relationships and psychotherapy* (pp. 315–328). New York: Springer Publishing Company.

Index

About the Author

Ofer Zur, PhD, is a licensed psychologist, instructor, forensic and ethics consultant, and expert witness in private psychotherapy practice in Sonoma, California. He is the director of the Zur Institute, which offers innovative and challenging continuing education online for psychologists, social workers, and counselors. His teaching in the United States and abroad as well as his writing focuses on ethics, critical thinking, boundaries, dual relationships, and the creation of managed-care-free private practices. For many years he taught at graduate schools, including the California School of Professional Psychology in Alameda and the California Institute of Integral Studies in San Francisco. His books include *Dual Relationships and Psychotherapy* (2002, coedited with Arnold Lazarus), *HIPAA Compliance Kit* (2005), and *The Complete Fee-for-Service Private Practice Handbook* (2005).